FOREVER STRONG COOKBOOK

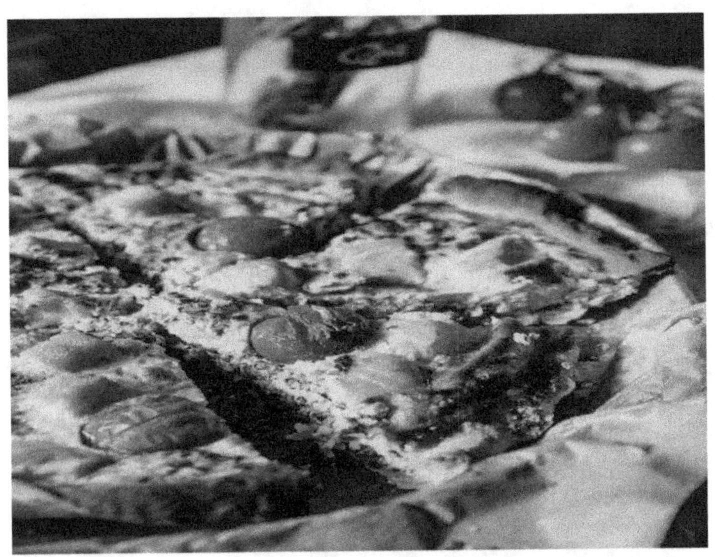

COMPREHENSIVE SCIENCE-BASED STRATEGY OF AGING WELL WITH OVER 80 DELICIOUS, NUTRITIOUS AND HEALTHY RECIPES.

ANNA SULLIVAN

Table of Contents

Introduction

Welcome to the "Forever Strong Cookbook," a gastronomic adventure that aims to change the way you think about aging and eating. We hope to lay the groundwork for an amazing journey into science-based nutrition and its tremendous influence on age-defying wellness in this introduction.

We honor each and every one of our valued readers' distinct ambitions and objectives. Our wide and vibrant audience includes baby boomers, Generation X, fitness enthusiasts, nutrition and wellness specialists, young folks planning for the future, those who are worried about appearance, and health enthusiasts. This cookbook is specifically designed for these individuals.

The "Forever Strong Cookbook" is centered around the combination of cutting-edge scientific knowledge and culinary expertise. We go into great detail on how eating well can help you stay youthful and vibrant. Learn the importance of antioxidants, the function that critical nutrients play, and the secrets of superfoods. With this knowledge, you'll be able to take charge of your own age-defying path.

We recognize that you're looking for a permanent change in addition to tasty meals. Our cookbook is a doorway to a day when you feel and look your best all the time. These recipes will enable you to:

Utilize nutrient-dense foods to help your body feel renewed.

Adopt a wellness-focused mindset that goes beyond fads and diets.

Enjoy the pure delight of indulging in delectable meals while staying well.

Discover the techniques for tastefully decelerating the aging process.

Ensure that your adolescent enthusiasm becomes a lifetime friend in the future.

The "Forever Strong Cookbook" is your guide to a timeless and vivid version of yourself; it's more than just a cookbook. We welcome you to explore every recipe, savor every page, and savor the knowledge that will enable you to achieve age-defying wellness as you set off on your gastronomic adventure. Welcome to a world where eating is the secret to staying young for all time.

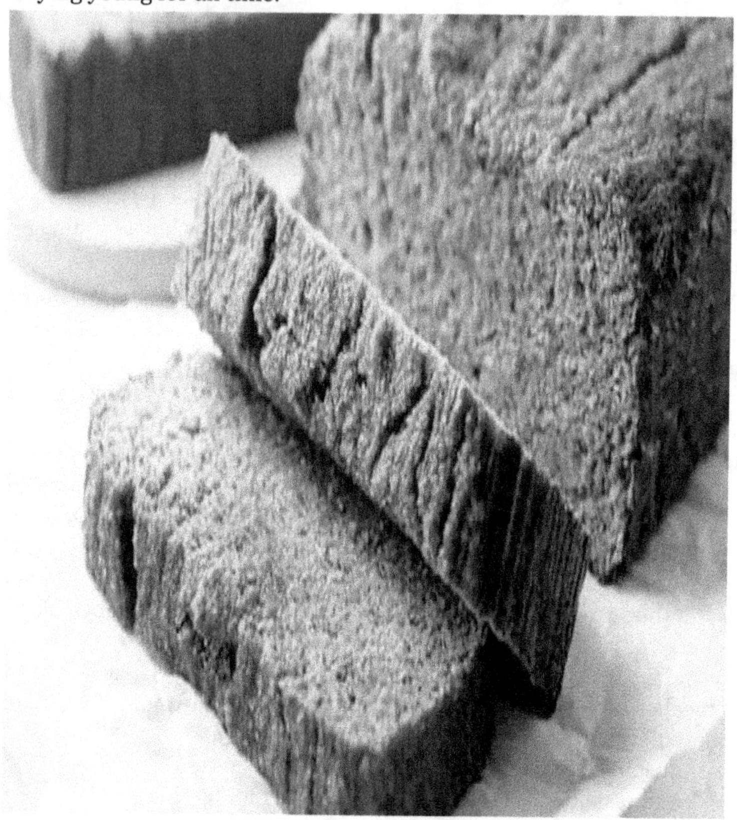

Chapter One

The Science of Youthful Nutrition

The search for the fountain of youth has gained prominence in a society where people are always trying to live longer and be more energetic. But rather than looking for fabled springs or enchanted concoctions, science and nutrition provide the solutions. This chapter explores the complex link between what we eat and how gracefully we age, delving into the principles of age-defying diet.

Exploring the Foundations of Age-Defying Nutrition

The first step in achieving young nutrition is comprehending the basic laws that control the aging process. Yes, we really are what we consume. Nutrition is more than simply filling our bellies; it's about giving our bodies the fundamental components they need to age with maximum health. We shall examine the scientific bases of the practice of young nutrition in this part.

Our bodies go through a number of intricate biochemical changes as we become older. It is essential to comprehend the science underlying these changes in order to create a diet that promotes vitality and longevity. The nutrients we eat can impact the aging process, from hormone changes to cellular deterioration. This information enables us to make educated nutrition decisions, paving the way for a more vibrant and healthy future.

Understanding the Impact of Dieting and Ageing

Diet is more than just a nutrition issue; it's a powerful instrument that may slow down or speed up the aging process. Every food we eat and beverage we consume affects how our bodies work, which has an effect on both our interior and external health. In this part, we set out to learn how our dietary choices might accelerate or decelerate the aging process.

Our general health can be significantly impacted by the decisions we make about the food that is on our plates. This chapter delves into the direct correlation between nutrition and aging, addressing subjects including inflammation, oxidative stress, and hormone regulation. Here, we solve the puzzles of how specific foods and eating habits might help maintain youthful vitality.

The Role of Antioxidants, Nutrients, and Superfoods

Antioxidants, minerals, and superfoods are the vivid paint brushes that give life and energy to the masterpiece of youthful nutrition, if diet is the canvas. This section explores the function of these vital elements in our nutritional repertoire and how they might help us withstand the passing of time.

Antioxidants are essential for shielding our cells from damage because of their extraordinary capacity to scavenge dangerous free radicals. From vital vitamins to trace minerals, nutrients are the building blocks of a diet that is well-balanced and promotes longevity. Furthermore, superfoods—nature's powerhouses of substances that promote health—give us an added advantage in our fight to age gracefully.

As we read through this chapter, we will get an understanding of the science underlying young people's nutrition as well as useful advice and ideas that we can use in our everyday lives. The quest for an age-defying diet is a realistic, scientific route to a longer, healthier, and more energetic life, not a fantastical undertaking. Greetings from the realm of young nourishment supported by science - a voyage towards a more optimistic and youthful future.

Chapter Two

Setting the Stage for Forever Youthful Living

Setting the scene for a lifetime of young living is essential as we go towards the region of everlasting vitality. We will look at the concrete actions that lead to this amazing journey in this chapter.

Assessing Your Current Diet and Health Goals

It's important to take stock of our situation before we throw ourselves into the art of living a youthful existence. The first vital step toward transformation is realizing where our nutrition and health are right now. We will walk you through the process of self-evaluation in this part, assisting you in assessing your objectives, health markers, and eating habits.

A thorough evaluation of your present circumstances is the compass that will direct your path, regardless of whether you're beginning from scratch or want to optimize your current diet plan. We'll go over how to monitor your daily consumption, assess any nutritional inadequacies, and pinpoint areas that want improvement. Equipped with this self-awareness, you'll be more capable of setting off on a path towards your own ideal of a youthful existence.

Embracing a Mindset for Lifelong Wellness

It's not just about what's on your plate—you also need to think positively to live a youthful life. It is impossible to overstate the influence that our thinking has on how we go on our path to lifetime wellbeing. We shall explore the mental side of the ageless living equation in this part.

Our beliefs about aging, diet, and health have a significant impact on the decisions we make. We'll delve into the idea of a "forever youthful" attitude, realizing that optimism and tenacity may fuel our dedication to a full life. On your journey to eternal youth, you'll learn how to stay motivated and get beyond typical mental obstacles.

Tips for Planning and Organizing Your Meals

You know what they say: "Failing to plan is planning to fail." Your meals are the foundation of your formative years, thus preparation and organization are essential. This section offers helpful hints and techniques for establishing meal plans that complement your health objectives.

We'll provide tips on how to make the process more effective and pleasurable, from grocery shopping to dinner preparation. You'll discover how to create balanced meals, manage portion sizes, and master the art of including those age-defying superfoods in your regular diet. You will be more capable of providing your body with the nutrition it needs for a lifetime of health if you have access to these useful tools.

We laid the foundation for the life-changing path to perpetual youth in this chapter. By taking stock of your current situation, adopting an optimistic outlook, and becoming an expert at meal planning, you'll be ready to go forward with assurance. You're on your way to realizing the road that leads to eternal vitality.

Chapter Three

Breakfasts for a Vibrant Start

It's true what they say—"breakfast is the most important meal of the day"—especially if we want to practice living young. We examine the science and art of creating breakfasts that provide the foundation for a day full of vigor and energy in this chapter.

Nutrient-Packed Morning Recipes to Kickstart Your Day

Breakfast is the first chance to provide your body the vital nutrients it needs to function at its peak, acting as a wake-up call. We've gathered a wealth of nutrient-dense breakfast meals in this area that will not only entice your palate but also fuel your body.

You may choose from protein-rich omelets loaded with vital amino acids and antioxidant-rich smoothie bowls bursting with vivid hues. Every recipe is thoughtfully crafted to provide you the energy to tackle the day by adding a boost of vigor to your morning routine.

1. Title: Superfood Breakfast Smoothie

Description: A powerhouse of nutrients to energize your morning.

Serving Size: 1 large glass

Prep Time: 5 minutes

Cooking Time: 0 minutes

Ingredients:

- 1 cup kale or spinach
- 1/2 ripe banana

- 1/2 cup mixed berries (e.g., blueberries, raspberries)
- 1 tablespoon chia seeds
- 1 cup unsweetened almond milk
- 1 tablespoon honey (optional)

Instructions:

1. Place kale or spinach, banana, mixed berries, chia seeds, and almond milk in a blender.
2. Blend until smooth.
3. Add honey if desired for sweetness.
4. Pour into a glass and enjoy your nutrient-packed superfood smoothie.

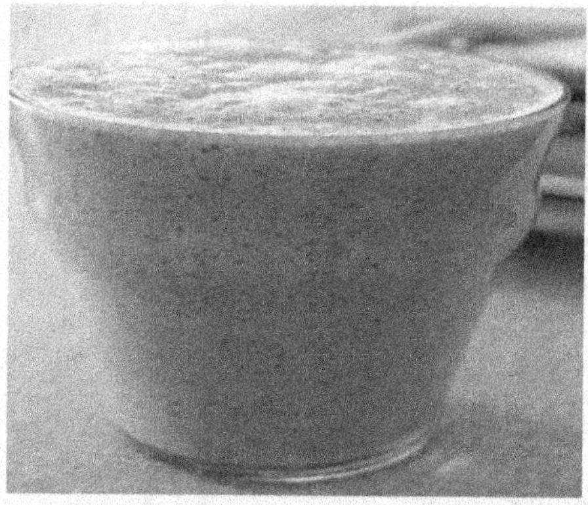

2. Title: Quinoa and Chia Seed Breakfast Bowl

Description: A protein and fiber-rich breakfast to fuel your day.

Serving Size: 1 bowl

Prep Time: 10 minutes

Cooking Time: 15 minutes

Ingredients:

- 1/2 cup cooked quinoa
- 1 tablespoon chia seeds
- 1/4 cup Greek yogurt
- 1/2 cup fresh mixed fruit (e.g., sliced strawberries, kiwi)
- 1 tablespoon almond butter
- A drizzle of honey

Instructions:

1. Cook quinoa according to package instructions and let it cool.
2. In a bowl, combine quinoa and chia seeds.
3. Top with Greek yogurt and fresh mixed fruit.
4. Drizzle with almond butter and honey.
5. Enjoy your quinoa and chia seed breakfast bowl.

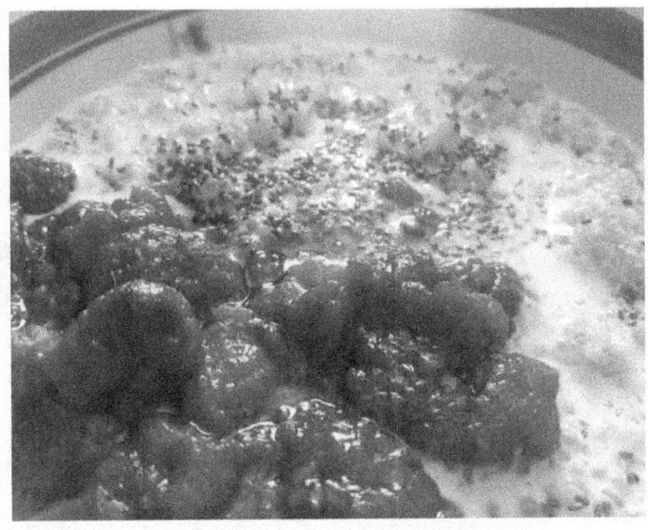

3. **Title: Avocado and Spinach Breakfast Wrap**

Description: A green-packed wrap for a morning nutrient boost.

Serving Size: 1 wrap

Prep Time: 10 minutes

Cooking Time: 5 minutes

Ingredients:

- 1 whole-grain tortilla
- 1/2 ripe avocado, mashed
- 1 cup fresh spinach leaves
- 2 eggs, scrambled
- Salt and pepper to taste
- Salsa for drizzling (optional)

Instructions:

1. Scramble the eggs in a pan, seasoning with salt and pepper.
2. Warm the tortilla in a separate pan.
3. Spread mashed avocado on the tortilla.
4. Add fresh spinach and scrambled eggs.
5. Drizzle with salsa if desired.
6. Fold into a wrap and enjoy your avocado and spinach breakfast wrap.

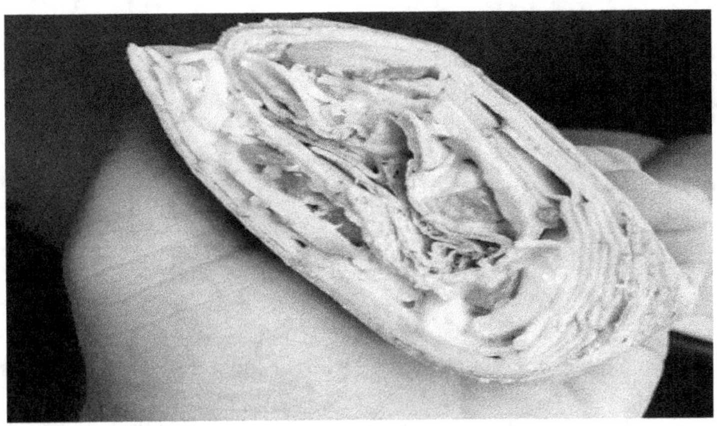

4. Title: Sweet Potato and Kale Breakfast Hash

Description: This hearty and nutritious Sweet Potato and Kale Breakfast Hash is the perfect way to start your day. Packed with sweet potatoes, kale, and eggs, it's a wholesome breakfast that provides the energy and nutrients you need to tackle the morning ahead. This dish is not only delicious but also a celebration of vibrant flavors and health-conscious choices.

Serving Size: 2 servings

Prep Time: 10 minutes

Cooking Time: 20 minutes

Ingredients:

- 2 small sweet potatoes, peeled and diced into small cubes
- 2 tablespoons olive oil
- 1/2 onion, finely chopped

- 2 cloves garlic, minced
- 2 cups kale, stems removed and chopped
- 1/2 teaspoon paprika
- Salt and pepper to taste
- 4 large eggs
- Chopped fresh parsley for garnish (optional)

Instructions:

1. Heat 1 tablespoon of olive oil in a large skillet over medium-high heat.
2. Add the diced sweet potatoes to the skillet. Spread them out in a single layer, allowing them to cook without stirring for a few minutes. This helps them become crisp.
3. Stir the sweet potatoes and continue cooking, occasionally stirring, until they are tender and slightly browned, approximately 10-12 minutes. You can cover the skillet to help them cook faster. Once done, transfer the sweet potatoes to a plate.
4. In the same skillet, add the remaining 1 tablespoon of olive oil and the chopped onion. Sauté the onion until it becomes translucent, about 3 minutes.
5. Add the minced garlic and cook for an additional 30 seconds, or until fragrant.
6. Stir in the chopped kale and cook until it wilts and becomes tender, approximately 5 minutes.
7. Return the cooked sweet potatoes to the skillet, then sprinkle with paprika, salt, and pepper. Stir to combine all the ingredients.
8. Create four wells or indentations in the hash. Crack an egg into each well.
9. Cover the skillet and cook until the egg whites are set but the yolks are still slightly runny, which should take about 5-7 minutes. If you prefer your eggs more well-done, cook them a little longer.
10. Sprinkle with chopped fresh parsley for garnish if desired.
11. Serve your Sweet Potato and Kale Breakfast Hash hot, dividing it into two portions. Enjoy your wholesome and satisfying breakfast!

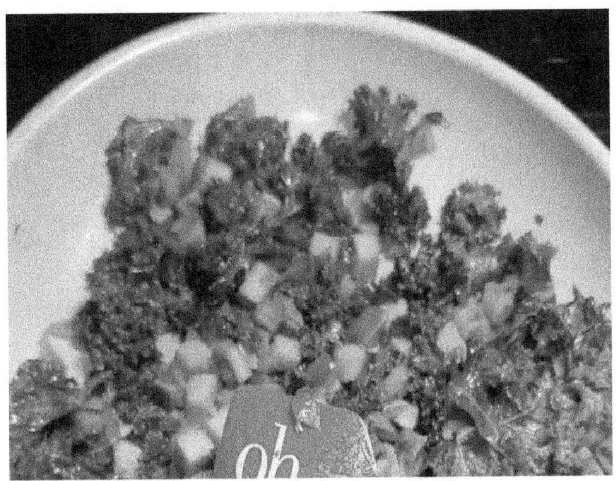

Options for Quick and Convenient Breakfasts

Convenience frequently influences our food choices in our fast-paced society. However, leading a healthy lifestyle should not be forfeited in the name of time restrictions. The breakfast selections in this area are designed to be quick and easy to fit into even the busiest schedules.

We'll go into the practice of making breakfast the night before for a hassle-free morning: overnight oats. We'll also explore the world of grab-and-go alternatives to make sure that, despite how busy you are during the day, you never skip breakfast.

1. Title: Grab-and-Go Breakfast Burrito

Description: A portable and protein-packed breakfast to fuel your day.

Serving Size: 1 burrito

Prep Time: 5 minutes

Cooking Time: 5 minutes

Ingredients:

- 1 large whole-grain tortilla
- 2 eggs, scrambled
- 1/4 cup black beans (canned, drained, and rinsed)
- 2 tablespoons salsa
- 1/4 cup shredded cheese
- Salt and pepper to taste

Instructions:

1. Place the tortilla on a flat surface.
2. Spread scrambled eggs, black beans, salsa, and shredded cheese down the center.
3. Season with salt and pepper.
4. Fold the sides of the tortilla, then roll it up tightly.
5. Microwave for about 30 seconds to melt the cheese.
6. Enjoy your grab-and-go breakfast burrito.

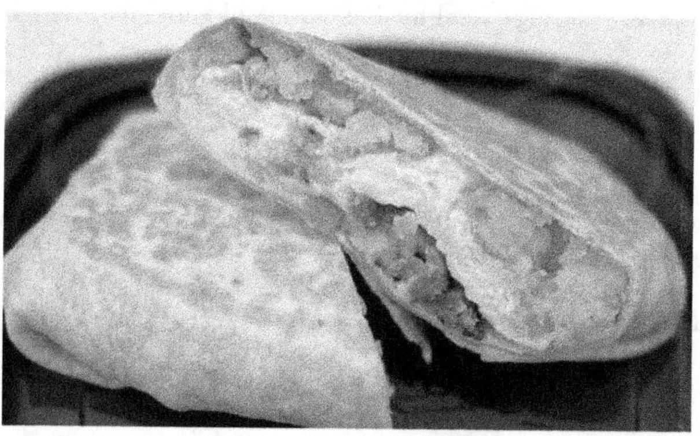

2. Overnight Oats

Description: A no-cook breakfast that's ready when you wake up.

Serving Size: 1 serving

Prep Time: 5 minutes

Cooking Time: 0 minutes

Ingredients:

- 1/2 cup rolled oats
- 1 cup milk (or milk alternative)
- 1 tablespoon honey
- 1/2 cup mixed berries
- 1 tablespoon chopped nuts (e.g., almonds, walnuts)

Instructions:

1. In a jar or bowl, combine rolled oats, milk, and honey.
2. Stir well and refrigerate overnight.
3. In the morning, top with mixed berries and chopped nuts.
4. Enjoy your convenient overnight oats.

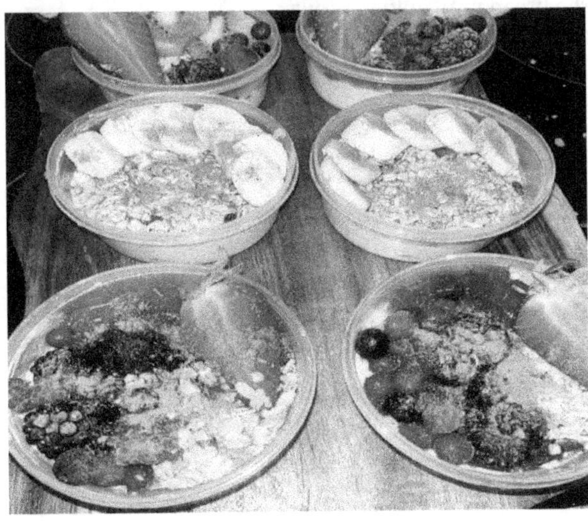

3. Title: Peanut Butter and Banana Toast

Description: A simple, yet satisfying breakfast that takes minutes to prepare.

Serving Size: 2 slices of toast

Prep Time: 5 minutes

Cooking Time: 0 minutes

Ingredients:

- 2 slices of whole-grain bread
- 2 tablespoons peanut butter
- 1 banana, sliced
- Honey for drizzling (optional)

Instructions:

1. Toast the bread until golden brown.
2. Spread peanut butter on each slice.
3. Top with banana slices.
4. Drizzle honey if desired.
5. Enjoy your peanut butter and banana toast.

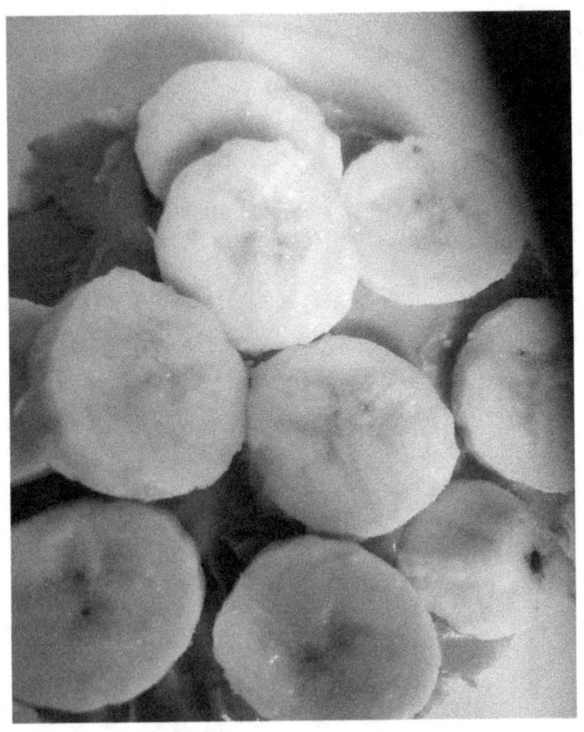

4. Title: Greek Yogurt Parfait

Description: A quick and customizable breakfast with layers of goodness.

Serving Size: 1 parfait

Prep Time: 5 minutes

Cooking Time: 0 minutes

Ingredients:

- 1 cup Greek yogurt
- 1/4 cup granola

- 1/2 cup mixed berries
- Honey for drizzling (optional)

Instructions:

1. In a glass or bowl, layer Greek yogurt, granola, and mixed berries.
2. Drizzle honey if desired.
3. Repeat the layers.
4. Enjoy your quick and delightful Greek yogurt parfait.

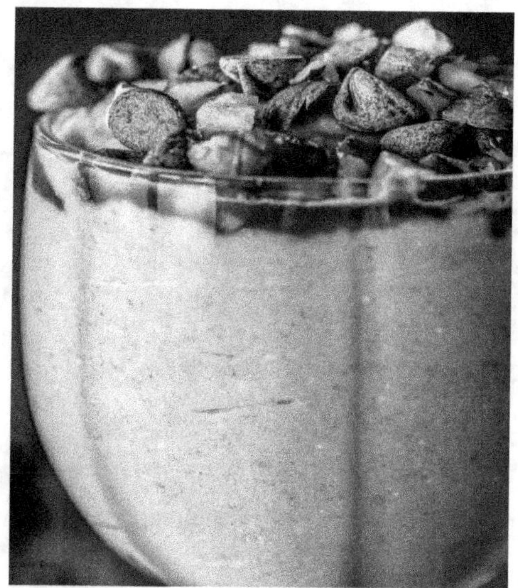

5. Title: Breakfast Smoothie in a Jar

Description: A portable, nutritious smoothie you can prepare the night before.

Serving Size: 1 jar

Prep Time: 5 minutes

Cooking Time: 0 minutes

Ingredients:

- 1/2 cup rolled oats
- 1/2 cup Greek yogurt
- 1/2 cup mixed berries
- 1 tablespoon chia seeds
- 1 cup almond milk
- 1 tablespoon honey (optional)

Instructions:

1. In a jar, layer rolled oats, Greek yogurt, mixed berries, chia seeds, and honey (if desired).
2. Pour almond milk over the ingredients.
3. Seal the jar and refrigerate overnight.
4. In the morning, give it a good shake and enjoy your breakfast smoothie on the go.

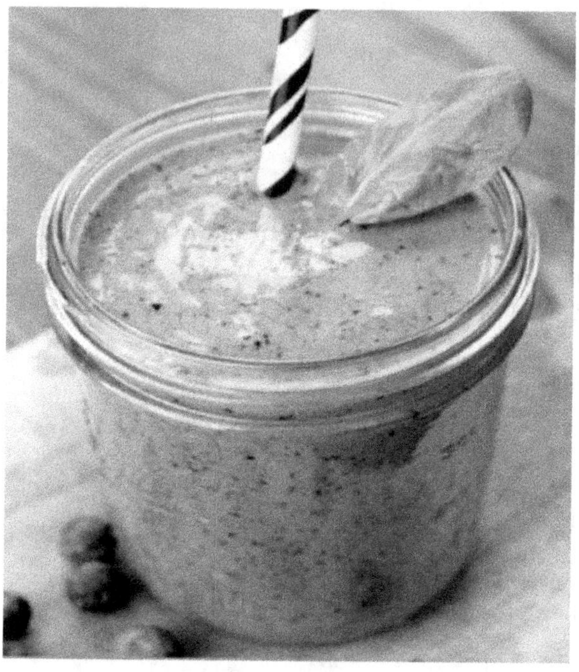

These quick and convenient breakfast recipes are perfect for hectic mornings. From breakfast burritos to overnight oats and simple toasts, these options ensure you get a nutritious start to your day without sacrificing precious time.

Write at least 5 Breakfasts for different Dietary preferences each recipe should include Title brief description or backstory serving size prep time & cooking time ingredients (clearly listed) and step by step instructions

Breakfasts for Different Dietary Preferences

We are aware that when it comes to food decisions, one size does not fit all. Whether you're a strict vegetarian, a carnivore in need of protein, or you adhere to a certain diet, we have breakfast alternatives to suit your needs. This section explores many dietary patterns through a culinary trip.

You can discover options that follow your nutritional guidelines, such as substantial breakfast burritos and plant-based smoothie bowls. Every dish has been carefully created to guarantee that you may have a tasty and nourishing start to your day, no matter what diet you follow.

1. Title: Vegan Berry Smoothie Bowl

Description: A plant-based and vibrant breakfast packed with antioxidants.

Serving Size: 1 bowl

Prep Time: 5 minutes

Cooking Time: 0 minutes

Ingredients:

- 1 cup mixed berries (strawberries, blueberries, raspberries)
- 1 ripe banana
- 1/2 cup almond milk
- 1 tablespoon chia seeds
- 1/4 cup granola
- Maple syrup for drizzling (optional)

Instructions:

1. Blend mixed berries, banana, and almond milk until smooth.
2. Pour the smoothie into a bowl.
3. Top with chia seeds, granola, and a drizzle of maple syrup, if desired.
4. Enjoy your vegan berry smoothie bowl.

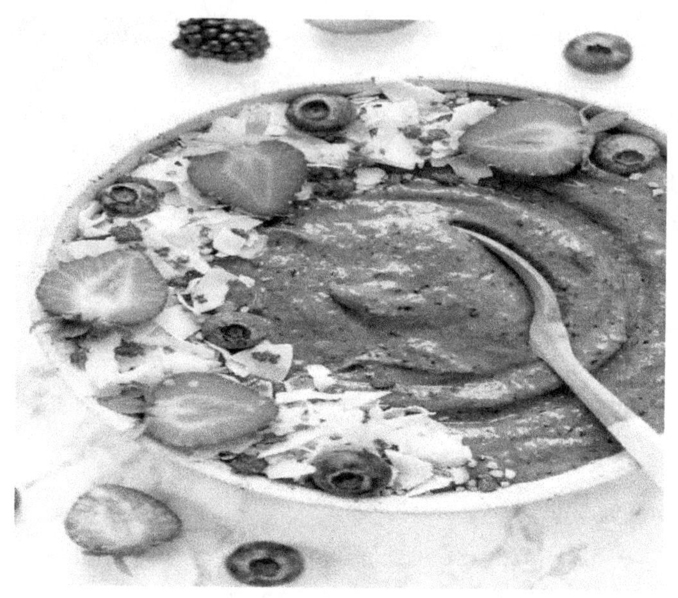

2. Title: High-Protein Egg and Spinach Breakfast

Description: A protein-packed breakfast suitable for those following a high-protein diet.

Serving Size: 1 serving

Prep Time: 10 minutes

Cooking Time: 10 minutes

Ingredients:

- 2 eggs
- 1 cup fresh spinach leaves

- 1/4 cup diced tomatoes
- 1/4 cup diced onions
- 1/4 cup shredded cheese
- Salt and pepper to taste

Instructions:

1. In a pan, sauté diced tomatoes and onions until soft.
2. Add fresh spinach and cook until wilted.
3. Whisk eggs, season with salt and pepper, and pour over the vegetables.
4. Scramble until eggs are cooked.
5. Top with shredded cheese.
6. Enjoy your high-protein egg and spinach breakfast.

3. Title: Gluten-Free Banana Pancakes

Description: A gluten-free breakfast option for those with dietary restrictions.

Serving Size: 2-3 pancakes

Prep Time: 10 minutes

Cooking Time: 10 minutes

Ingredients:

- 2 ripe bananas, mashed
- 2 eggs
- 1/2 cup almond flour
- 1/2 teaspoon baking powder
- 1/2 teaspoon vanilla extract
- A pinch of salt

Instructions:

1. In a bowl, combine mashed bananas, eggs, almond flour, baking powder, vanilla extract, and a pinch of salt.
2. Heat a non-stick pan over medium heat and lightly grease with cooking spray or oil.
3. Pour small portions of the batter onto the pan to form pancakes.
4. Cook until bubbles appear on the surface, then flip and cook the other side until golden brown.
5. Serve your gluten-free banana pancakes with your favorite toppings.

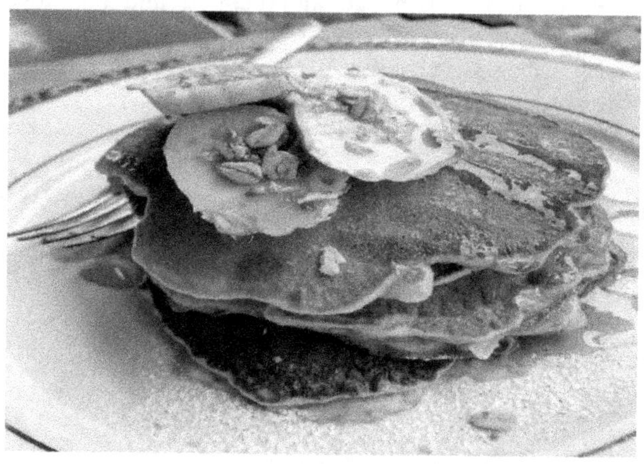

4. Title: Keto Avocado and Bacon Egg Cups

Description: A low-carb, high-fat breakfast perfect for those following a ketogenic diet.

Serving Size: 2 servings (2 egg cups each)

Prep Time: 10 minutes

Cooking Time: 15 minutes

Ingredients:

- 2 eggs
- 1 avocado, halved and pitted
- 2 slices of bacon
- Salt and pepper to taste
- Chopped chives for garnish (optional)

Instructions:

1. Preheat the oven to 350°F (175°C).
2. Cut a small slice from the bottom of each avocado half to create a stable base.
3. Place avocados in a baking dish.
4. Crack an egg into each avocado half.
5. Wrap each avocado with a slice of bacon.
6. Bake for about 15 minutes or until eggs are set to your liking.
7. Season with salt and pepper and garnish with chives, if desired.
8. Enjoy your keto avocado and bacon egg cups.

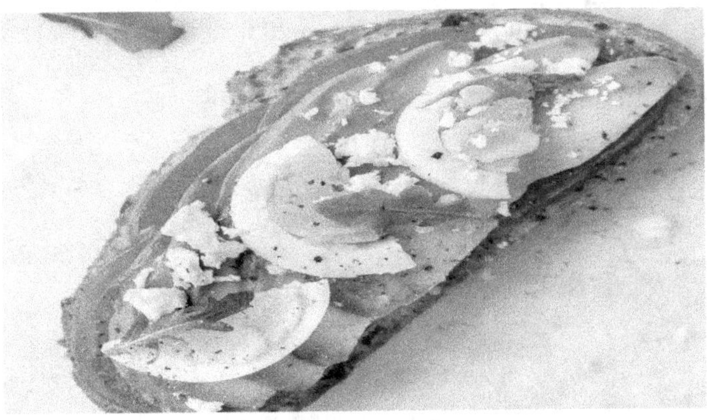

5. Title: Nut-Free Apple Cinnamon Oatmeal

Description: A nut-free breakfast for those with nut allergies or sensitivities.

Serving Size: 1 serving

Prep Time: 5 minutes

Cooking Time: 5 minutes

Ingredients:

- 1/2 cup rolled oats
- 1 cup milk (or milk alternative)
- 1 apple, peeled, cored, and diced
- 1/2 teaspoon cinnamon
- 1 tablespoon honey
- A pinch of salt

Instructions:

1. In a saucepan, combine rolled oats, milk, diced apple, cinnamon, honey, and a pinch of salt.
2. Cook over medium heat, stirring, until the oats are tender and the mixture thickens.
3. Serve your nut-free apple cinnamon oatmeal.

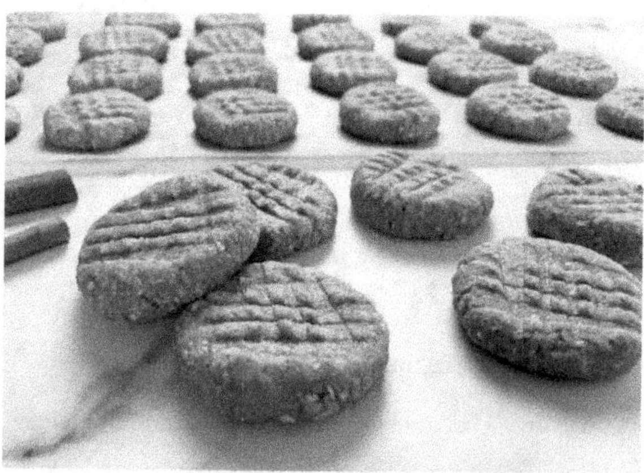

These breakfast recipes cater to various dietary preferences, ensuring that everyone can enjoy a delicious and satisfying morning meal. Whether you're vegan, high-protein, gluten-free, following a keto diet, or nut-free, these recipes have you covered.

In this chapter, we set the stage for a vibrant day with breakfast choices that nourish your body and tantalize your taste buds. With nutrient-packed recipes, quick and convenient options, and choices for various dietary preferences, you'll be equipped to kickstart your day with the vitality and energy you need to thrive. Breakfast is no longer just a meal; it's the cornerstone of your journey towards a lifetime of youthful living.

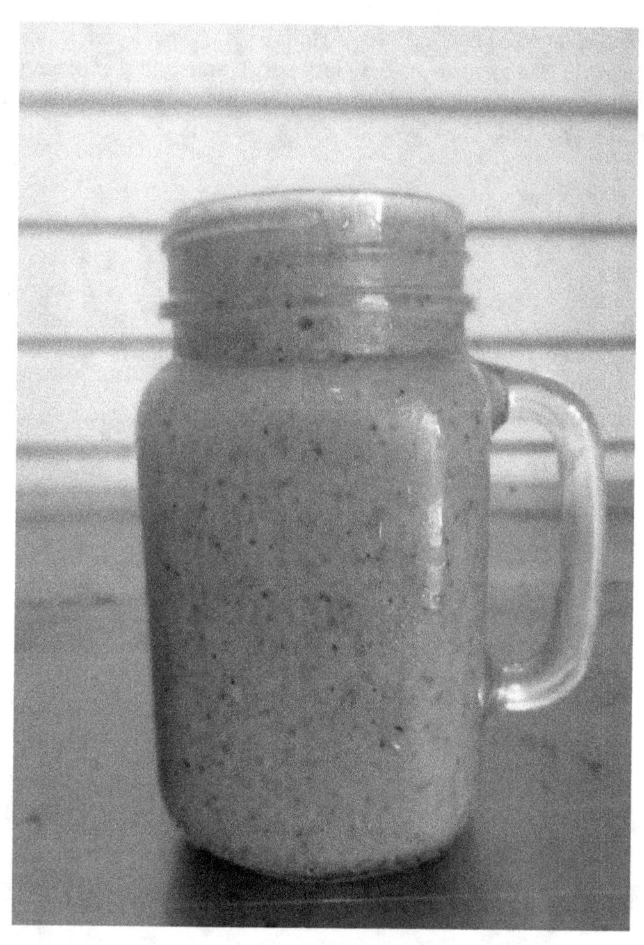

Chapter Four

Lunchtime Rejuvenation

Our demand for a noon meal that nourishes our body and soul peaks at the same time as the sun. This chapter explores the realm of midday rejuvenation, offering you stimulating meal options that will give you the energy and purpose to tackle the day.

Energizing Lunch Ideas to Sustain Your Day

Lunch is an important part of your day, not just a time to pause and recharge. Now is the perfect moment to refuel, refocus, and re energize. This area offers a tonne of lunch options that will energize your body and mind, so you can perform at your peak all afternoon.

Our invigorating lunch options include a wide range of flavors and textures, from substantial soups that warm your soul to power-packed salads loaded with minerals. Every meal is painstakingly prepared to provide you the precise ratio of macronutrients as well as the vital vitamins and minerals you require to take on the day's demands.

1. **Title: Quinoa and Chickpea Salad with Lemon-Tahini Dressing**

Description: A protein-packed salad with a zesty dressing to keep you energized.

Serving Size: 2 servings

Prep Time: 15 minutes

Cooking Time: 15 minutes

Ingredients:

- 1 cup cooked quinoa
- 1 can (15 oz) chickpeas, drained and rinsed
- 1 cup cherry tomatoes, halved
- 1 cucumber, diced
- 1/4 cup red onion, finely chopped
- 1/4 cup fresh parsley, chopped
- 2 tablespoons tahini
- Juice of 1 lemon
- 2 tablespoons olive oil
- Salt and pepper to taste

Instructions:

1. In a large bowl, combine quinoa, chickpeas, cherry tomatoes, cucumber, red onion, and fresh parsley.
2. In a separate bowl, whisk together tahini, lemon juice, and olive oil to make the dressing.
3. Pour the dressing over the salad and toss to coat.
4. Season with salt and pepper to taste.
5. Divide into servings and enjoy your energizing quinoa and chickpea salad.

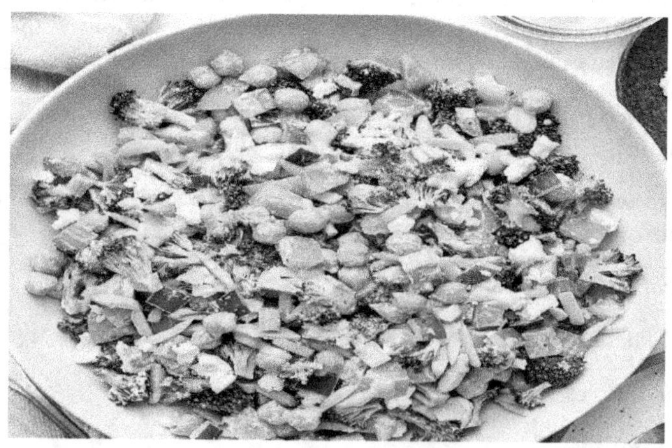

2. **Title: Sushi-Inspired Rice Bowl**

Description: A deconstructed sushi bowl that's as flavorful as it is energizing.

Serving Size: 2 servings

Prep Time: 20 minutes

Cooking Time: 0 minutes

Ingredients:

- 2 cups cooked sushi rice
- 1/2 pound sushi-grade raw salmon or tuna, thinly sliced
- 1/2 avocado, sliced
- 1/2 cucumber, thinly sliced
- 1/4 cup pickled ginger
- 2 tablespoons soy sauce
- Wasabi and sesame seeds for garnish (optional)

Instructions:

1. Divide the sushi rice into two bowls.
2. Arrange slices of raw fish, avocado, and cucumber on top of the rice.
3. Drizzle soy sauce over the bowls.
4. Garnish with pickled ginger and, if desired, wasabi and sesame seeds.
5. Enjoy your sushi-inspired rice bowl.

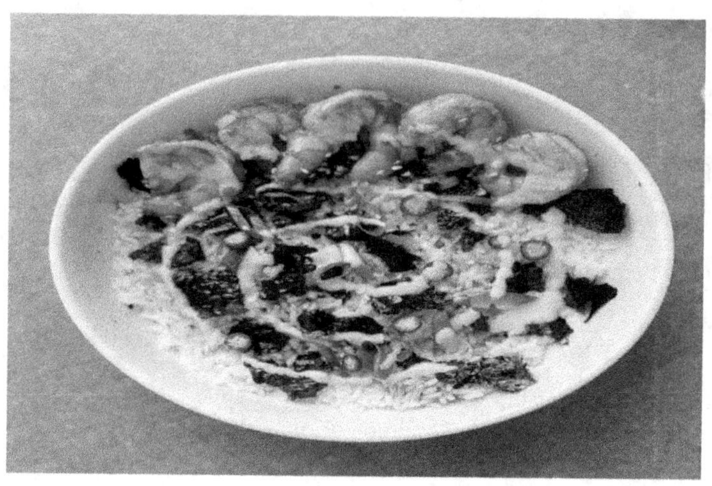

3. Title: Spinach and Quinoa Stuffed Bell Peppers

Description: A balanced and energizing lunch, stuffed with vibrant flavors.

Serving Size: 2 servings

Prep Time: 20 minutes

Cooking Time: 25 minutes

Ingredients:

- 2 bell peppers, any color
- 1 cup cooked quinoa
- 1 cup baby spinach, chopped
- 1/2 cup cherry tomatoes, diced
- 1/4 cup feta cheese, crumbled
- 2 tablespoons olive oil

- Salt and pepper to taste

Instructions:

1. Preheat the oven to 375°F (190°C).
2. Cut the tops off the bell peppers and remove the seeds.
3. In a bowl, mix quinoa, chopped baby spinach, cherry tomatoes, and feta cheese.
4. Stuff the bell peppers with the quinoa mixture.
5. Drizzle with olive oil and season with salt and pepper.
6. Place the stuffed peppers in a baking dish and bake for 25 minutes or until the peppers are tender.
7. Enjoy your spinach and quinoa stuffed bell peppers.

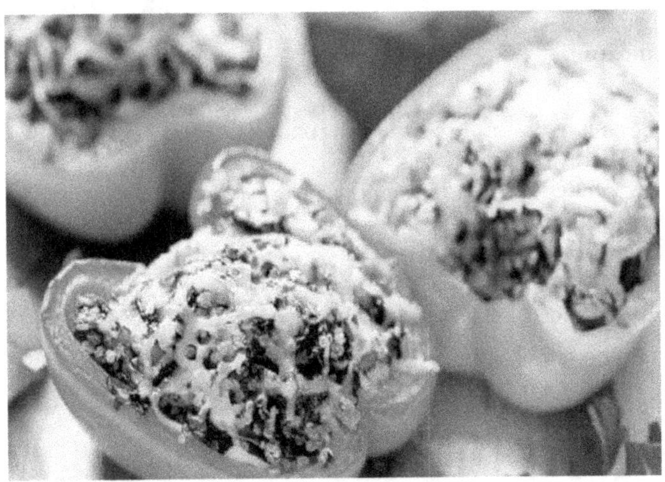

4. Title: Chicken and Avocado Wrap

Description: A protein-rich and portable lunch to keep you going.

Serving Size: 2 wraps

Prep Time: 15 minutes

Cooking Time: 10 minutes

Ingredients:

- 2 boneless, skinless chicken breasts
- 1 tablespoon olive oil
- 1/2 teaspoon paprika
- 1/2 teaspoon garlic powder
- Salt and pepper to taste
- 2 whole-grain tortillas
- 1 avocado, sliced
- 1 cup mixed greens
- Greek yogurt or hummus for spreading

Instructions:

1. Season chicken breasts with paprika, garlic powder, salt, and pepper.
2. Heat olive oil in a pan and cook the chicken until no longer pink inside (about 5 minutes per side).
3. Slice the cooked chicken.
4. Lay out the tortillas and spread Greek yogurt or hummus on each.
5. Layer sliced avocado, mixed greens, and sliced chicken on each tortilla.
6. Roll up the tortillas and cut in half.
7. Enjoy your chicken and avocado wraps.

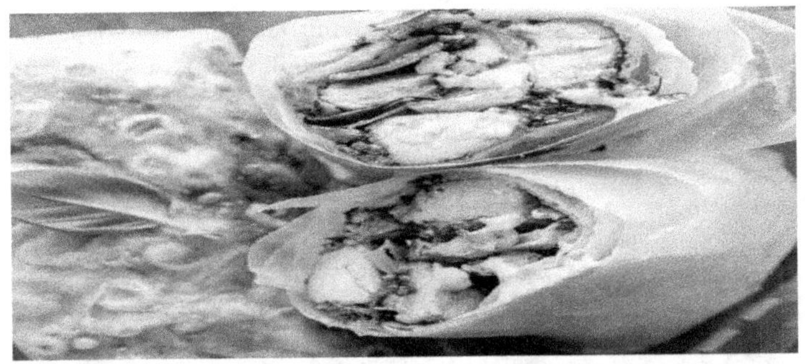

5. Title: Lentil and Vegetable Soup

Description: A hearty and warming soup to sustain your energy throughout the day.

Serving Size: 4 servings

Prep Time: 15 minutes

Cooking Time: 30 minutes

Ingredients:

- 1 cup green or brown lentils, rinsed
- 1 carrot, diced
- 1 celery stalk, diced
- 1 onion, chopped
- 2 cloves garlic, minced
- 6 cups vegetable broth
- 1 teaspoon cumin
- 1/2 teaspoon turmeric
- Salt and pepper to taste

Instructions:

1. In a large pot, sauté onions, garlic, carrots, and celery until soft.

2. Add lentils, vegetable broth, cumin, turmeric, salt, and pepper.
3. Bring to a boil, then reduce to a simmer and cook for 25-30 minutes or until lentils are tender.
4. Serve your lentil and vegetable soup hot and enjoy.

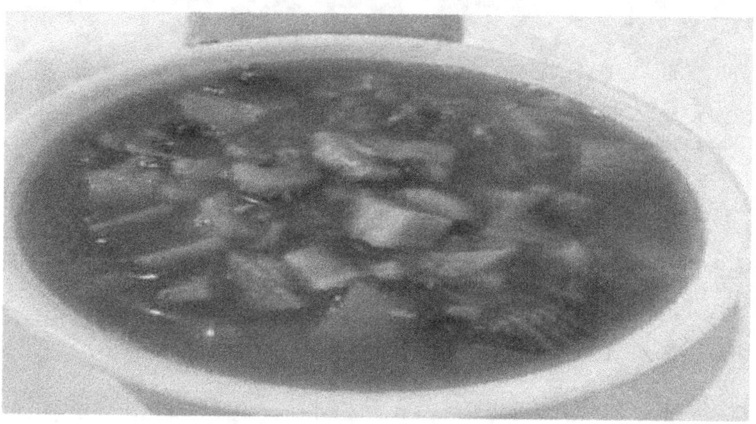

These energizing lunch ideas are designed to keep you nourished and sustained throughout your busy day, whether you're at work, school, or on the go. From salads and wraps to hearty soups, these recipes offer a variety of flavors and textures to please your palate while providing the energy you need.

Balanced and Satisfying Midday Meals

A balanced lunch considers both your physical and emotional needs. This section of the chapter delves into the art of creating midday meals that fulfill your palate and make you feel happy and energized.

We'll walk you through the principles of creating lunchtime meals that balance proteins, healthy fats, and complex carbs. You'll find dishes that not only taste great but also support prolonged energy and satiety, so you can take on the remainder of your day with renewed enthusiasm.

1. **Mediterranean Quinoa Bowl**

Description: A well-balanced and satisfying lunch inspired by Mediterranean flavors.

Serving Size: 2 servings

Prep Time: 15 minutes

Cooking Time: 15 minutes

Ingredients:

- 1 cup cooked quinoa
- 1 can (15 oz) chickpeas, drained and rinsed
- 1 cucumber, diced
- 1 cup cherry tomatoes, halved
- 1/2 red onion, thinly sliced
- 1/4 cup Kalamata olives, pitted and sliced
- 1/4 cup crumbled feta cheese
- 2 tablespoons olive oil
- Juice of 1 lemon
- 1 teaspoon dried oregano
- Salt and pepper to taste

Instructions:

1. In a large bowl, combine quinoa, chickpeas, cucumber, cherry tomatoes, red onion, Kalamata olives, and feta cheese.
2. In a separate bowl, whisk together olive oil, lemon juice, dried oregano, salt, and pepper to make the dressing.
3. Pour the dressing over the salad and toss to combine.
4. Divide into servings and enjoy your Mediterranean quinoa bowl.

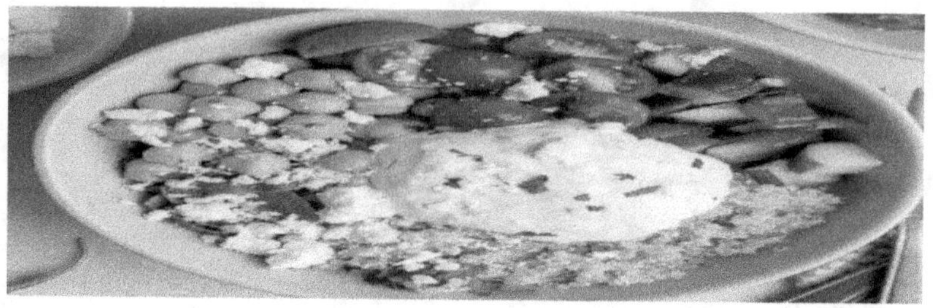

2. Title: Balanced Chicken and Vegetable Stir-Fry

Description: A stir-fry that combines protein and a variety of vegetables for a well-balanced meal.

Serving Size: 2 servings

Prep Time: 15 minutes

Cooking Time: 15 minutes

Ingredients:

- 2 boneless, skinless chicken breasts, cut into thin strips
- 2 tablespoons soy sauce
- 1 tablespoon olive oil
- 1 bell pepper, sliced
- 1 cup broccoli florets
- 1 carrot, sliced into matchsticks
- 1/2 cup snow peas
- 2 cloves garlic, minced
- 1/2 teaspoon ginger, grated
- Cooked brown rice or quinoa for serving

Instructions:

1. In a bowl, marinate chicken strips in soy sauce for about 10 minutes.
2. Heat olive oil in a large pan or wok over high heat.
3. Add marinated chicken and stir-fry until cooked through, then transfer to a plate.
4. In the same pan, add garlic and ginger, then add vegetables and stir-fry until crisp-tender.
5. Return the chicken to the pan and cook for an additional minute.
6. Serve the stir-fry over cooked brown rice or quinoa.
7. Enjoy your balanced chicken and vegetable stir-fry.

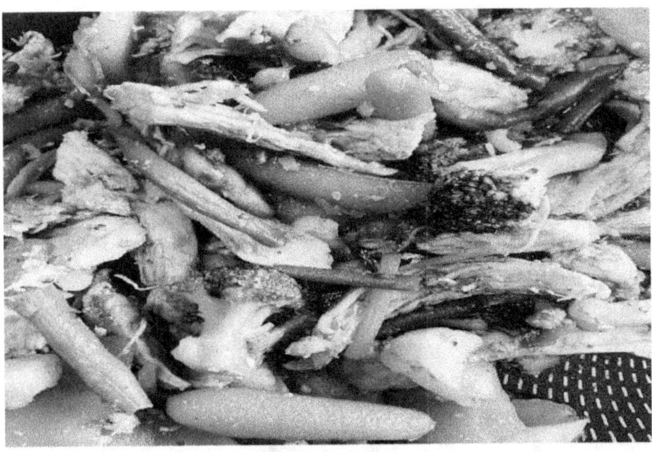

3. Salmon and Quinoa Stuffed Bell Peppers

Description: A balanced and satisfying meal featuring salmon and quinoa.

Serving Size: 2 servings

Prep Time: 20 minutes

Cooking Time: 30 minutes

Ingredients:

- 2 bell peppers, any color
- 2 salmon fillets
- 1 cup cooked quinoa
- 1 cup baby spinach, chopped
- 1/2 cup cherry tomatoes, diced
- 2 tablespoons olive oil
- Salt and pepper to taste

Instructions:

1. Preheat the oven to 375°F (190°C).
2. Cut the tops off the bell peppers and remove the seeds.
3. Brush salmon fillets with olive oil and season with salt and pepper.
4. Bake the salmon in the oven for about 20 minutes or until flaky.
5. In a bowl, combine quinoa, chopped baby spinach, and cherry tomatoes.
6. Stuff the bell peppers with the quinoa mixture.
7. Place baked salmon on top of the quinoa in the peppers.
8. Bake for an additional 10 minutes.
9. Enjoy your salmon and quinoa stuffed bell peppers.

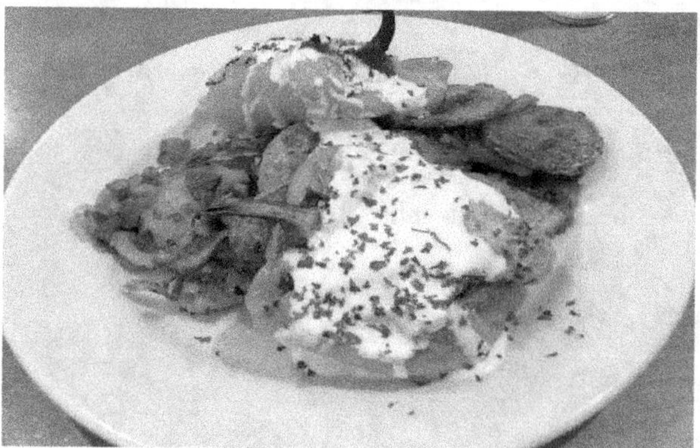

4. Title: Tofu and Veggie Thai Green Curry

Description: A balanced and satisfying Thai green curry with tofu and vegetables.

Serving Size: 2 servings

Prep Time: 15 minutes

Cooking Time: 20 minutes

Ingredients:

- 8 oz tofu, cubed
- 2 tablespoons green curry paste
- 1 can (14 oz) coconut milk
- 1 cup broccoli florets
- 1 carrot, sliced into thin rounds
- 1 red bell pepper, sliced
- 1 cup snow peas
- 2 tablespoons fish sauce or soy sauce (for a vegetarian version)
- Juice of 1 lime
- Fresh cilantro for garnish
- Cooked jasmine rice for serving

Instructions:

1. In a large skillet, heat the green curry paste until fragrant.
2. Add coconut milk and bring to a simmer.
3. Add tofu, broccoli, carrot, red bell pepper, and snow peas.
4. Cook until vegetables are tender and tofu is heated through.
5. Stir in fish sauce (or soy sauce) and lime juice.
6. Serve the curry over cooked jasmine rice.
7. Garnish with fresh cilantro.
8. Enjoy your tofu and veggie Thai green curry.

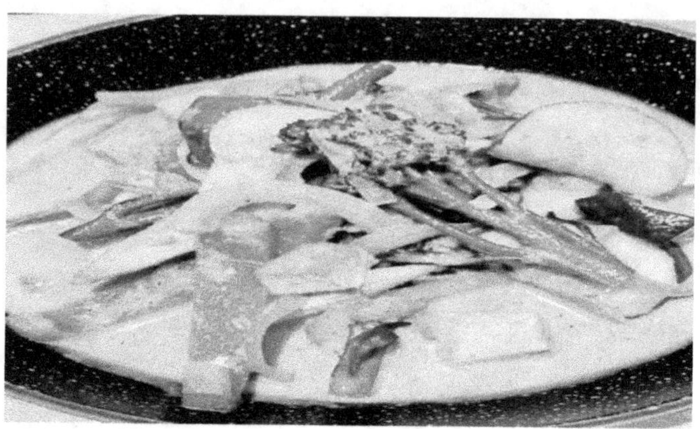

5. Title: Balanced Lentil and Quinoa Salad

Description: A protein-rich salad with lentils and quinoa for a balanced and satisfying meal.

Serving Size: 2 servings

Prep Time: 20 minutes

Cooking Time: 20 minutes

Ingredients:

- 1/2 cup green or brown lentils, rinsed
- 1/2 cup quinoa
- 2 cups water
- 1 cup cherry tomatoes, halved
- 1 cucumber, diced
- 1/4 cup red onion, finely chopped
- 1/4 cup fresh parsley, chopped
- Juice of 1 lemon
- 2 tablespoons olive oil

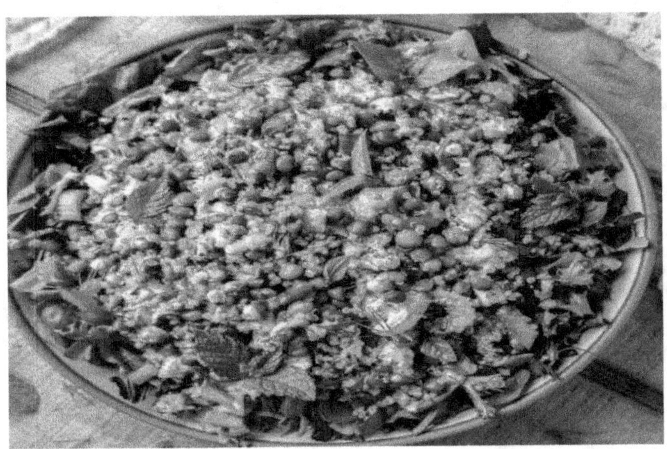

Vegan, Low-Carb, and Gluten-Free Lunch Options

We acknowledge that dietary choices and limitations are as varied as the individuals who adhere to them. Here, we accommodate a variety of dietary requirements with a selection of lunch alternatives for vegans, low-carbohydrate diets, and gluten-sensitive people.

Our selection of plant-based lunch options is a celebration of tastes and ingredients. They don't depend on animal products and offer an abundance of minerals. Our selection of low-carb lunch options will provide you satisfying substitutes that won't make you feel like you're gaining weight. We also have products that are free of gluten but still have a great taste and texture for people who require them.

1. Title: Vegan Cauliflower Rice Stir-Fry

Description: A low-carb and gluten-free stir-fry with cauliflower rice as the base.

Serving Size: 2 servings

Prep Time: 15 minutes

Cooking Time: 15 minutes

Ingredients:

- 1 small head of cauliflower
- 2 tablespoons olive oil
- 1 cup broccoli florets
- 1 cup sliced bell peppers (various colors)
- 1 cup snap peas
- 1 carrot, julienned
- 1/4 cup sliced scallions
- 1/4 cup gluten-free tamari sauce (or soy sauce)
- 1 tablespoon rice vinegar
- 1 teaspoon sesame oil
- Salt and pepper to taste

Instructions:

1. Cut the cauliflower into florets and pulse in a food processor until it resembles rice.
2. Heat olive oil in a large pan or wok over medium heat.
3. Add cauliflower rice and sauté for 3-4 minutes until tender.
4. In the same pan, add broccoli, bell peppers, snap peas, carrot, and scallions. Stir-fry for another 5-7 minutes until vegetables are tender.
5. In a small bowl, whisk together tamari sauce, rice vinegar, sesame oil, salt, and pepper.
6. Pour the sauce over the stir-fry and cook for an additional 2 minutes.
7. Serve your vegan cauliflower rice stir-fry.

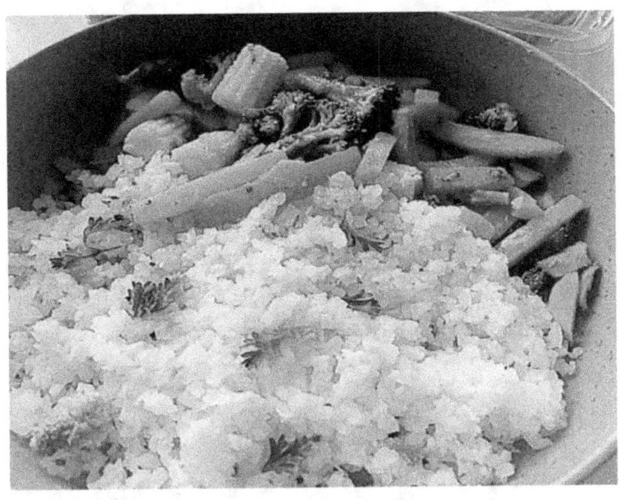

2. Title: Zucchini Noodles with Pesto

Description: A low-carb, gluten-free lunch with zucchini noodles and a flavorful pesto sauce.

Serving Size: 2 servings

Prep Time: 15 minutes

Cooking Time: 5 minutes

Ingredients:

- 4 medium zucchinis
- 1 cup fresh basil leaves
- 1/4 cup pine nuts
- 2 cloves garlic
- 1/4 cup nutritional yeast (for a cheesy flavor)
- 1/4 cup olive oil
- Juice of 1 lemon
- Salt and pepper to taste

Instructions:

1. Use a spiralizer to create zucchini noodles from the zucchinis.
2. In a food processor, combine fresh basil, pine nuts, garlic, nutritional yeast, olive oil, lemon juice, salt, and pepper. Blend into a pesto sauce.
3. Toss the zucchini noodles with the pesto sauce until well coated.
4. Serve your zucchini noodles with pesto.

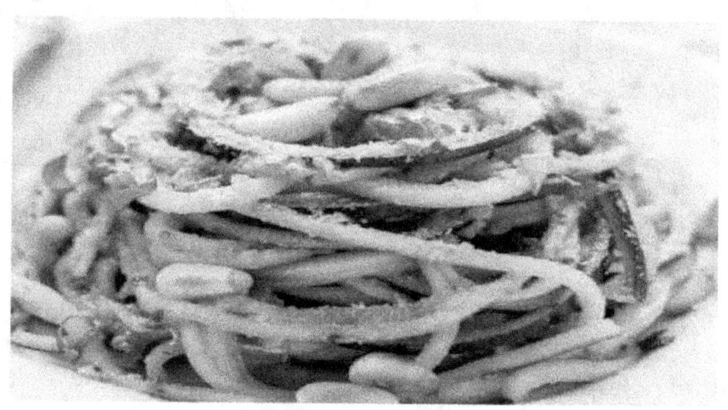

3. Vegan Mediterranean Salad

Description: A fresh and colorful salad inspired by Mediterranean cuisine.

Serving Size: 2 servings

Prep Time: 15 minutes

Cooking Time: 0 minutes

Ingredients:

- 1 cup cooked quinoa
- 1 can (15 oz) chickpeas, drained and rinsed
- 1 cucumber, diced

- 1 cup cherry tomatoes, halved
- 1/4 cup red onion, finely chopped
- 1/4 cup Kalamata olives, pitted and sliced
- 1/4 cup fresh parsley, chopped
- Juice of 1 lemon
- 2 tablespoons olive oil
- Salt and pepper to taste

Instructions:

1. In a large bowl, combine cooked quinoa, chickpeas, cucumber, cherry tomatoes, red onion, Kalamata olives, and fresh parsley.
2. In a separate bowl, whisk together lemon juice, olive oil, salt, and pepper to make the dressing.
3. Pour the dressing over the salad and toss to coat.
4. Divide into servings and enjoy your vegan Mediterranean salad.

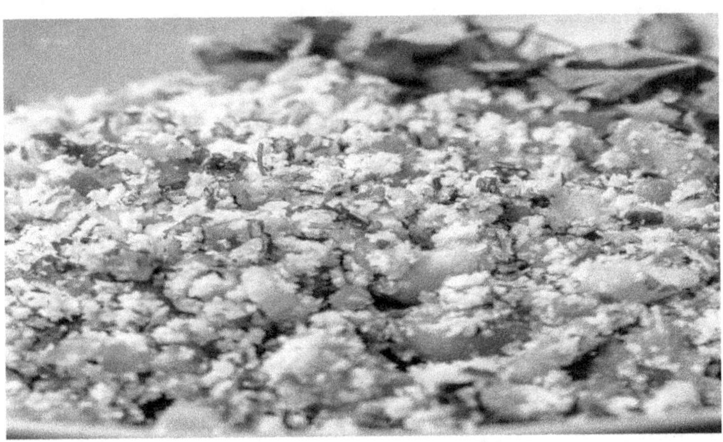

4. Title: Vegan Avocado and Black Bean Salad

Description: A refreshing and low-carb salad with creamy avocado and protein-packed black beans.

Serving Size: 2 servings

Prep Time: 15 minutes

Cooking Time: 0 minutes

Ingredients:

- 2 avocados, diced
- 1 can (15 oz) black beans, drained and rinsed
- 1 cup corn kernels (fresh or frozen, thawed)
- 1/4 cup red onion, finely chopped
- 1/4 cup fresh cilantro, chopped
- Juice of 1 lime
- Salt and pepper to taste

Instructions:

1. In a large bowl, combine diced avocados, black beans, corn, red onion, and cilantro.
2. Squeeze lime juice over the salad and gently toss.
3. Season with salt and pepper to taste.
4. Serve your vegan avocado and black bean salad.

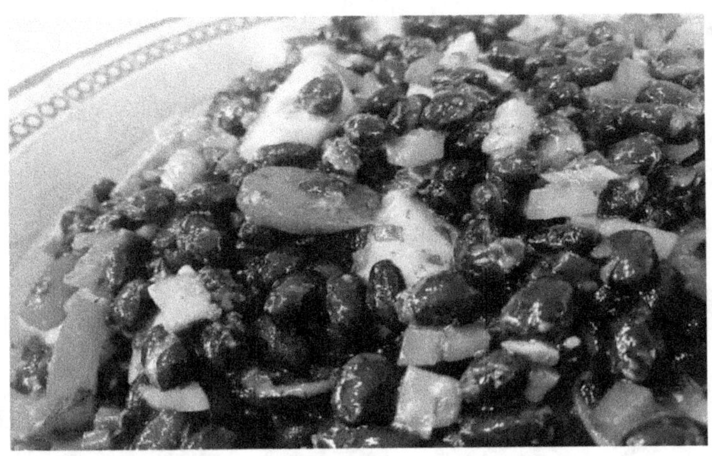

5. Title: Vegan Broccoli and "Cheese" Soup

Description: A warm and comforting soup that's vegan and gluten-free, with a cheesy flavor.

Serving Size: 4 servings

Prep Time: 15 minutes

Cooking Time: 25 minutes

Ingredients:

- 4 cups broccoli florets
- 1 potato, peeled and diced
- 1 carrot, peeled and diced
- 1 onion, chopped
- 2 cloves garlic, minced
- 4 cups vegetable broth
- 1 cup unsweetened almond milk (or any plant-based milk)
- 1/2 cup nutritional yeast
- 1/2 teaspoon turmeric
- Salt and pepper to taste

Instructions:

1. In a large pot, combine broccoli, potato, carrot, onion, garlic, and vegetable broth.
2. Bring to a boil, then reduce heat, cover, and simmer for 20 minutes or until vegetables are tender.
3. Use an immersion blender to puree the soup until smooth.
4. Stir in almond milk, nutritional yeast, turmeric, salt, and pepper.
5. Heat for an additional 5 minutes.
6. Serve your vegan broccoli and "cheese" soup.

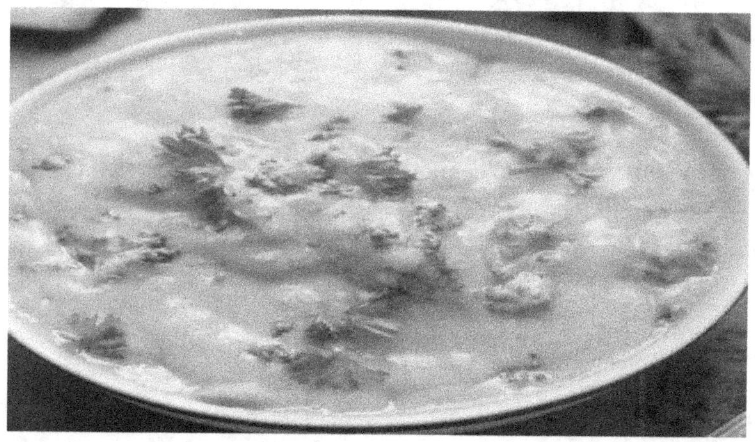

These vegan, low-carb, and gluten-free lunch options offer a variety of flavors and textures while keeping your dietary preferences and restrictions in mind. Whether you're in the mood for a stir-fry, noodles, a refreshing salad, or a comforting soup, these recipes have you covered.

This chapter takes us on a midday rejuvenation journey, converting a daily requirement into a time of hydration and energy. With alternatives for a variety of dietary requirements, healthy midday meals, and creative lunch ideas, your lunch turns into a critical source of inspiration for the rest of your day's excursions. Lunch is now a moment to shine and refresh, not just a break.

Chapter Five

Dinner Delights for Timeless Elegance

The evening promises gastronomic grandeur as the sun sets, transforming supper from a simple meal into a work of art. This chapter delves into the world of "Dinner Delights for Timeless Elegance," where delicious evening meals come with a plethora of health advantages.

Evening Meals Infused with Flavor and Health Benefits

Dinner ought to be a celebration of life's basic joys, a symphony of flavor and nutrition. This section delves deeply into the artistry of creating evening meals that are not only delicious to eat but also good for your health.

Our recipes emphasize the use of seasonal foods, flavorful herbs and spices, and cooking methods that enhance tastes while retaining the nutritional value of each ingredient. We present you a menu of dinners that are full of flavor and health, ranging from heart-friendly selections to foods that promote good digestion and general energy.

1. Title: Grilled Salmon with Lemon-Dill Quinoa

Description: A heart-healthy meal that combines the richness of salmon with the freshness of lemon and dill.

Serving Size: 2 servings

Prep Time: 15 minutes

Cooking Time: 20 minutes

Ingredients:

- 2 salmon fillets
- 1 cup quinoa

- 2 cups water
- Zest and juice of 1 lemon
- 2 tablespoons fresh dill, chopped
- 2 tablespoons olive oil
- Salt and pepper to taste

Instructions:

1. Season the salmon fillets with lemon zest, half of the lemon juice, dill, 1 tablespoon of olive oil, salt, and pepper.
2. Preheat a grill or grill pan and cook the salmon for about 4-5 minutes on each side or until cooked to your liking.
3. In a saucepan, bring water to a boil, then add quinoa. Reduce heat, cover, and simmer for about 15 minutes or until quinoa is cooked.
4. Fluff the cooked quinoa with a fork, and stir in the remaining lemon juice and olive oil.
5. Serve the grilled salmon over a bed of lemon-dill quinoa.

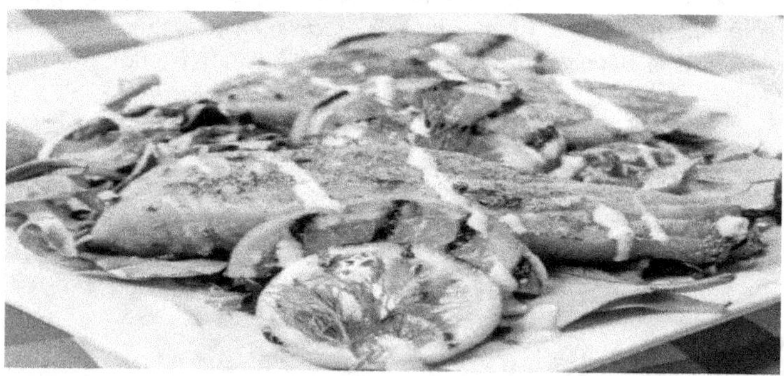

2. Title: Roasted Vegetable and Chickpea Salad

Description: A fiber-rich salad that bursts with the flavors of roasted vegetables and protein-packed chickpeas.

Serving Size: 4 servings

Prep Time: 15 minutes

Cooking Time: 30 minutes

Ingredients:

- 1 red bell pepper, sliced
- 1 yellow bell pepper, sliced
- 1 zucchini, sliced
- 1 red onion, sliced
- 1 can (15 oz) chickpeas, drained and rinsed
- 2 tablespoons olive oil
- 1 teaspoon paprika
- Salt and pepper to taste
- 4 cups mixed greens
- Balsamic vinaigrette for dressing

Instructions:

1. Preheat the oven to 400°F (200°C).
2. In a large bowl, toss the red and yellow bell peppers, zucchini, red onion, chickpeas, olive oil, paprika, salt, and pepper.
3. Spread the mixture on a baking sheet and roast for about 25-30 minutes until vegetables are tender and slightly caramelized.
4. Arrange mixed greens on serving plates.
5. Top with the roasted vegetable and chickpea mixture.
6. Drizzle with balsamic vinaigrette.
7. Enjoy your roasted vegetables and chickpea salad.

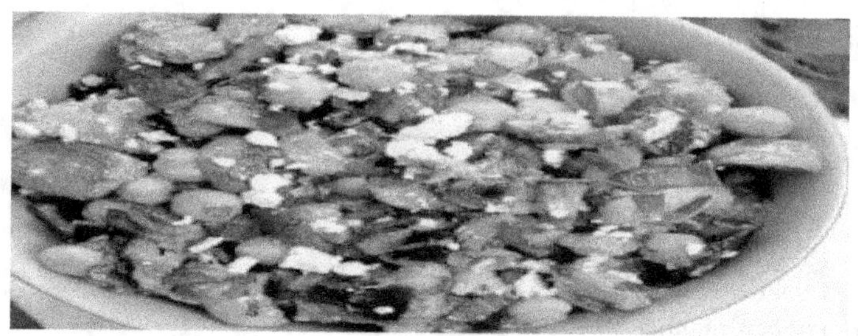

3. Title: Ginger-Garlic Tofu Stir-Fry

Description: A stir-fry bursting with the flavors of ginger and garlic, featuring protein-packed tofu.

Serving Size: 2 servings

Prep Time: 15 minutes

Cooking Time: 15 minutes

Ingredients:

- 8 oz extra-firm tofu, cubed
- 2 tablespoons soy sauce
- 1 tablespoon sesame oil
- 1 tablespoon rice vinegar
- 1 tablespoon fresh ginger, minced
- 2 cloves garlic, minced
- 1 red bell pepper, sliced
- 1 cup broccoli florets
- 1 cup snap peas
- Cooked brown rice for serving

Instructions:

1. In a bowl, marinate tofu cubes in soy sauce for about 10 minutes.
2. In a wok or large skillet, heat sesame oil over medium-high heat.

3. Add marinated tofu and stir-fry until browned.
4. Add ginger and garlic, and stir-fry for another minute.
5. Add red bell pepper, broccoli, and snap peas. Stir-fry until vegetables are crisp-tender.
6. Stir in rice vinegar.
7. Serve your ginger-garlic tofu stir-fry over cooked brown rice.

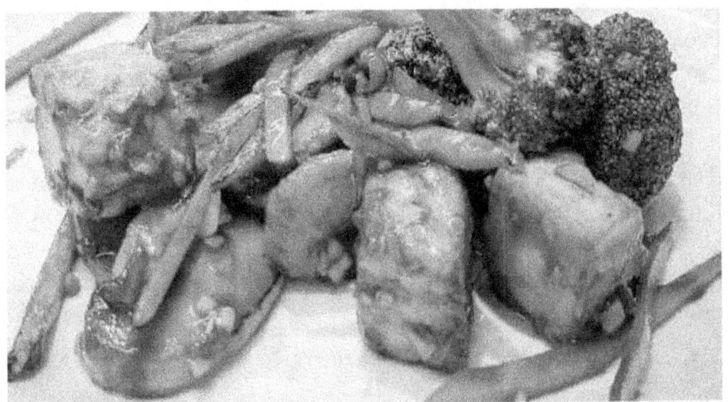

4. Title: Stuffed Bell Peppers with Quinoa and Black Beans

Description: A plant-based meal that combines the goodness of quinoa and black beans in vibrant bell peppers.

Serving Size: 4 servings

Prep Time: 20 minutes

Cooking Time: 45 minutes

Ingredients:

- 4 bell peppers, any color
- 1 cup cooked quinoa
- 1 can (15 oz) black beans, drained and rinsed
- 1 cup corn kernels (fresh or frozen, thawed)
- 1/4 cup red onion, finely chopped

- 1/4 cup fresh cilantro, chopped
- 1 teaspoon cumin
- Salt and pepper to taste
- 1 cup tomato sauce

Instructions:

1. Preheat the oven to 375°F (190°C).
2. Cut the tops off the bell peppers and remove the seeds.
3. In a large bowl, combine cooked quinoa, black beans, corn, red onion, cilantro, cumin, salt, and pepper.
4. Stuff the bell peppers with the quinoa and black bean mixture.
5. Place the stuffed peppers in a baking dish and pour tomato sauce over them.
6. Cover with foil and bake for about 35-40 minutes or until peppers are tender.
7. Enjoy your stuffed bell peppers with quinoa and black beans.

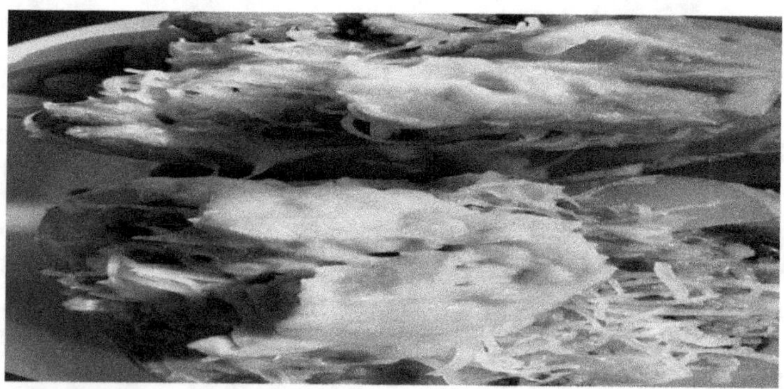

5. Title: Vegan Lentil Curry

Description: A flavorful and protein-rich curry with red lentils and a blend of spices.

Serving Size: 4 servings

Prep Time: 15 minutes

Cooking Time: 30 minutes

Ingredients:

- 1 cup red lentils, rinsed
- 1 onion, chopped
- 2 cloves garlic, minced
- 1 tablespoon fresh ginger, minced
- 1 can (14 oz) diced tomatoes
- 1 can (14 oz) coconut milk
- 1 tablespoon curry powder
- 1 teaspoon turmeric
- 1 teaspoon cumin
- Salt and pepper to taste
- Fresh cilantro for garnish
- Cooked basmati rice for serving

Instructions:

1. In a large pot, sauté onions, garlic, and ginger until softened.
2. Add lentils, diced tomatoes, coconut milk, curry powder, turmeric, cumin, salt, and pepper. Stir well.
3. Bring to a simmer, cover, and cook for about 20-25 minutes or until lentils are tender and the mixture has thickened.
4. Serve your vegan lentil curry over cooked basmati rice, garnished with fresh cilantro.

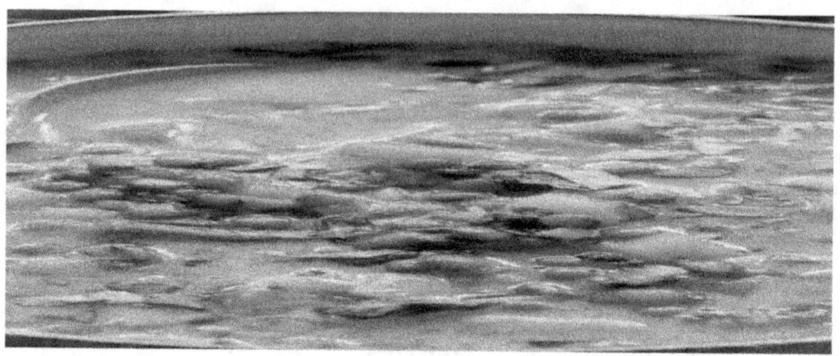

These evening meals not only tantalize the taste buds but also offer a variety of health benefits. From heart-healthy salmon to protein-packed tofu and fiber-rich salads, these recipes are perfect for a flavorful and nutritious dinner.

Special Dinner Recipes for Celebrations and Gatherings

Dinner is a time to celebrate significant occasions and spend happy moments with loved ones; it's more than just a daily habit. We provide a selection of meal dishes for celebrations and gatherings in this section of the chapter.

These dishes, which range from elegant main courses to rich desserts, are made with an additional dash of elegance and are ideal for birthdays, anniversaries, or any other special occasion you want to remember. Whether you're having a little family get-together or throwing a lavish party, these unique supper recipes will make the occasion elegant and delightful.

1. Title: Herb-Crusted Rack of Lamb

Description: A luxurious dish featuring tender rack of lamb with a flavorful herb crust.

Serving Size: 4 servings

Prep Time: 15 minutes

Cooking Time: 30 minutes

Ingredients:

- 2 racks of lamb (8 ribs each)
- 2 tablespoons Dijon mustard
- 2 cloves garlic, minced
- 2 tablespoons fresh rosemary, chopped
- 2 tablespoons fresh thyme, chopped
- 1 cup breadcrumbs
- Salt and pepper to taste
- Olive oil for searing

Instructions:

1. Preheat the oven to 425°F (220°C).
2. Season the racks of lamb with salt and pepper.
3. Heat olive oil in an ovenproof skillet. Sear the lamb racks on all sides until browned.
4. In a bowl, mix Dijon mustard, minced garlic, chopped rosemary, and chopped thyme.
5. Roll the seared lamb racks in the herb mixture to coat.
6. Roll the coated lamb racks in breadcrumbs.
7. Place the racks in the skillet and roast in the preheated oven for about 20 minutes or until they reach your desired level of doneness.
8. Slice the lamb into individual chops and serve.

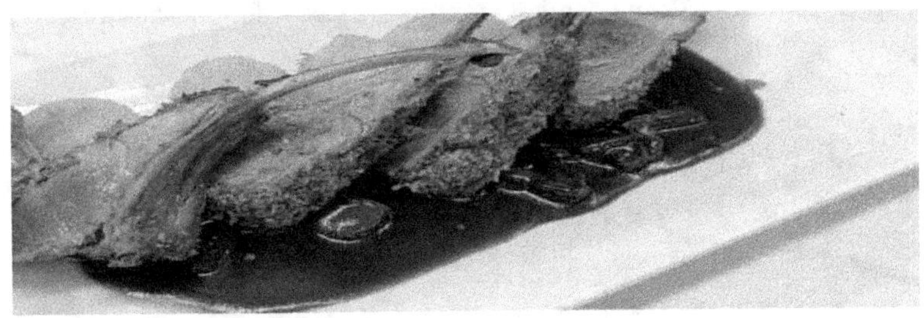

2. Title: Lobster and Shrimp Scampi

Description: A seafood delight featuring succulent lobster and shrimp in a garlicky white wine sauce.

Serving Size: 4 servings

Prep Time: 15 minutes

Cooking Time: 20 minutes

Ingredients:

- 4 lobster tails, split in half
- 1 pound large shrimp, peeled and deveined
- 4 cloves garlic, minced
- 1/4 cup fresh parsley, chopped
- 1/4 cup white wine
- 1/4 cup lemon juice
- 1/4 cup butter
- Salt and pepper to taste
- Cooked linguine or spaghetti for serving

Instructions:

1. In a large skillet, melt the butter over medium-high heat.
2. Add minced garlic and cook for about 1 minute.
3. Add lobster tails and shrimp and sauté until they turn pink and opaque.
4. Stir in white wine and lemon juice. Cook for an additional 2 minutes.
5. Toss in chopped parsley and season with salt and pepper.
6. Serve your lobster and shrimp scampi over cooked linguine or spaghetti.

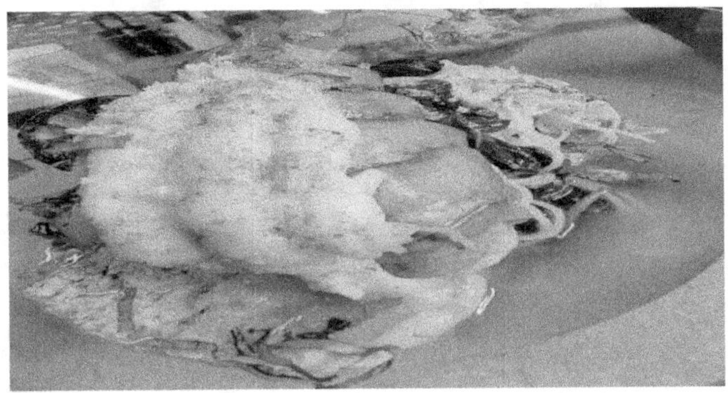

3. Title: Beef Wellington

Description: A classic and impressive dish featuring tender beef fillet encased in puff pastry.

Serving Size: 4 servings

Prep Time: 30 minutes

Cooking Time: 45 minutes

Ingredients:

- 1 1/2 pounds beef fillet
- 2 tablespoons olive oil
- 2 cloves garlic, minced
- 1 tablespoon Dijon mustard
- 1 package puff pastry sheets
- 4 slices prosciutto
- 1 egg (beaten, for egg wash)
- Salt and pepper to taste

Instructions:

1. Preheat the oven to 400°F (200°C).

2. Season the beef fillet with salt and pepper.
3. In a hot skillet, sear the beef fillet on all sides until browned.
4. Brush the fillet with Dijon mustard and let it cool.
5. Roll out the puff pastry sheets and lay prosciutto slices on them.
6. Place the beef fillet on the prosciutto and wrap it tightly in the puff pastry.
7. Brush with egg wash and bake for about 30-35 minutes or until the pastry is golden and the beef reaches your desired level of doneness.
8. Slice the beef Wellington and serve.

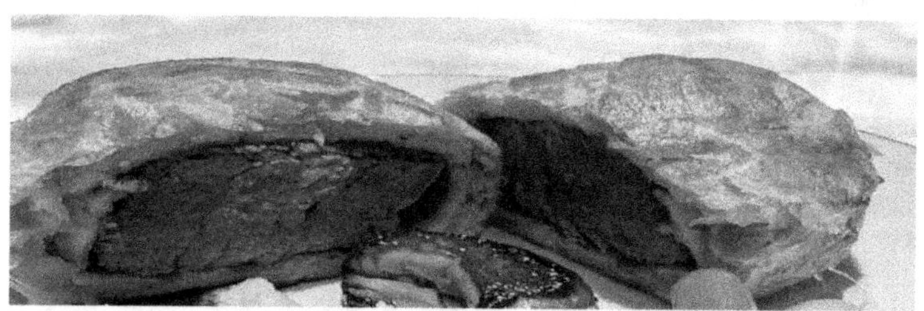

4. Title: Mushroom Risotto

Description: A creamy and comforting risotto loaded with earthy mushrooms.

Serving Size: 4 servings

Prep Time: 10 minutes

Cooking Time: 30 minutes

Ingredients:

- 1 1/2 cups Arborio rice
- 4 cups vegetable broth
- 1 cup white wine
- 2 cups mixed mushrooms (such as cremini, shiitake, and oyster), sliced

- 1 onion, finely chopped
- 2 cloves garlic, minced
- 2 tablespoons olive oil
- 1/2 cup grated Parmesan cheese
- Fresh thyme leaves for garnish
- Salt and pepper to taste

Instructions:

1. In a large pot, heat olive oil over medium heat. Add chopped onion and garlic and sauté until translucent.
2. Add Arborio rice and cook for 2 minutes, stirring.
3. Pour in white wine and cook until it's mostly absorbed.
4. Begin adding vegetable broth, one ladle at a time, stirring frequently until the liquid is absorbed before adding more.
5. In a separate pan, sauté the sliced mushrooms until they release their moisture and become tender.

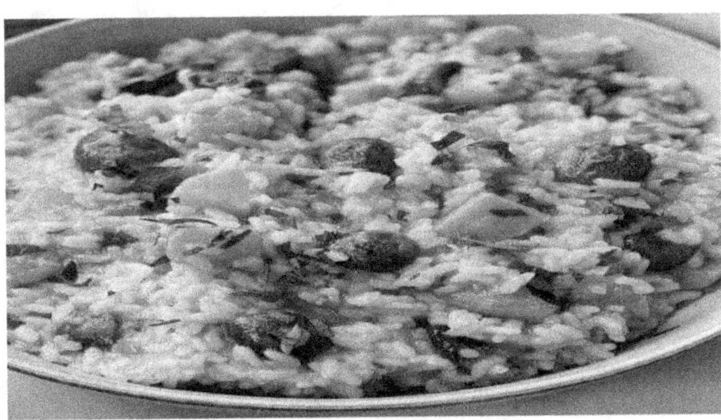

5. Title: Pomegranate Glazed Duck Breast

Description: An exquisite dish that combines the richness of duck with a sweet and tangy pomegranate glaze.

Serving Size: 4 servings

Prep Time: 15 minutes

Cooking Time: 25 minutes

Ingredients:

- 4 duck breast fillets
- 1 cup pomegranate juice
- 1/4 cup balsamic vinegar
- 1/4 cup honey
- 2 cloves garlic, minced
- Salt and pepper to taste
- Fresh pomegranate arils and fresh rosemary for garnish

Instructions:

1. Score the skin of the duck breasts in a crisscross pattern without cutting into the meat. Season with salt and pepper.
2. In a hot skillet, place the duck breasts skin side down and cook for about 5-7 minutes until the skin is crispy and browned. Flip and cook for an additional 3-5 minutes, or until the duck reaches your desired level of doneness. Remove from the skillet and let it rest.
3. In the same skillet, add minced garlic and sauté for about 1 minute.
4. Pour in pomegranate juice, balsamic vinegar, and honey. Bring to a simmer and cook until the sauce thickens.
5. Slice the duck breasts and drizzle with the pomegranate glaze.
6. Garnish with fresh pomegranate arils and rosemary.
7. Serve your pomegranate glazed duck breast for a truly special dinner.

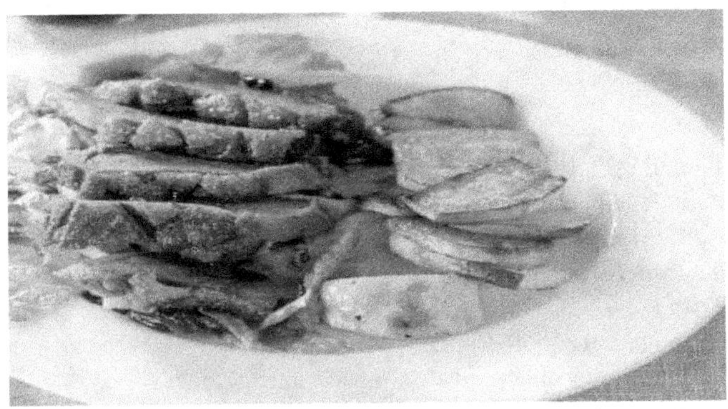

Dietary-Specific Dinner Options

We try to accommodate the wide range of dietary needs and preferences that we are aware of. We offer supper suggestions in this area that can accommodate different dietary requirements.

We provide a meal alternative for everyone, regardless of their dietary preferences—vegan, paleo, gluten-free, or just a pescatarian relishing the bounty of the sea. We make sure that everyone may enjoy the sophistication of a well-prepared evening meal with our diet-specific dishes.

This chapter honors the ageless grace of supper, where each mouthful is a culinary adventure and each dish is a nutritional masterpiece. Whether you're looking for dietary-specific solutions, a feast for a particular occasion, or health advantages, our dinner treats will make sure your evening meals are a monument to the skill of timeless flavor and culinary brilliance.

1. Title: Vegan Butternut Squash and Chickpea Curry

Description: A flavorful and satisfying vegan curry featuring butternut squash and protein-packed chickpeas.

Serving Size: 4 servings

Prep Time: 15 minutes

Cooking Time: 25 minutes

Ingredients:

- 1 small butternut squash, peeled, seeded, and diced
- 1 can (15 oz) chickpeas, drained and rinsed
- 1 onion, chopped
- 2 cloves garlic, minced
- 1 can (14 oz) diced tomatoes
- 1 can (14 oz) coconut milk
- 2 tablespoons curry powder
- 1 tablespoon olive oil
- Salt and pepper to taste
- Fresh cilantro for garnish
- Cooked basmati rice for serving

Instructions:

1. In a large pot, heat olive oil over medium heat. Add chopped onion and garlic and sauté until softened.
2. Add diced butternut squash and cook for about 5 minutes.
3. Stir in curry powder, salt, and pepper.
4. Add chickpeas, diced tomatoes, and coconut milk. Stir well.
5. Bring to a simmer, cover, and cook for about 15-20 minutes or until the butternut squash is tender.
6. Serve your vegan butternut squash and chickpea curry over cooked basmati rice, garnished with fresh cilantro.

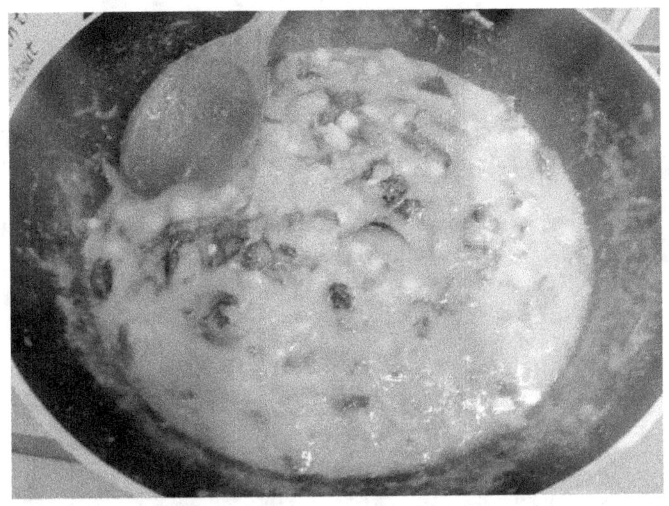

2. Title: Low-Carb Zucchini Noodles with Pesto

Description: A low-carb, gluten-free, and keto-friendly dinner featuring zucchini noodles with a flavorful pesto sauce.

Serving Size: 2 servings

Prep Time: 15 minutes

Cooking Time: 10 minutes

Ingredients:

- 4 medium zucchinis
- 1 cup fresh basil leaves
- 1/4 cup pine nuts
- 2 cloves garlic
- 1/4 cup nutritional yeast (for a cheesy flavor)
- 1/4 cup olive oil
- Juice of 1 lemon
- Salt and pepper to taste

Instructions:

1. Use a spiralizer to create zucchini noodles from the zucchinis.
2. In a food processor, combine fresh basil, pine nuts, garlic, nutritional yeast, olive oil, lemon juice, salt, and pepper. Blend into a pesto sauce.
3. Toss the zucchini noodles with the pesto sauce until well coated.
4. Serve your low-carb zucchini noodles with pesto.

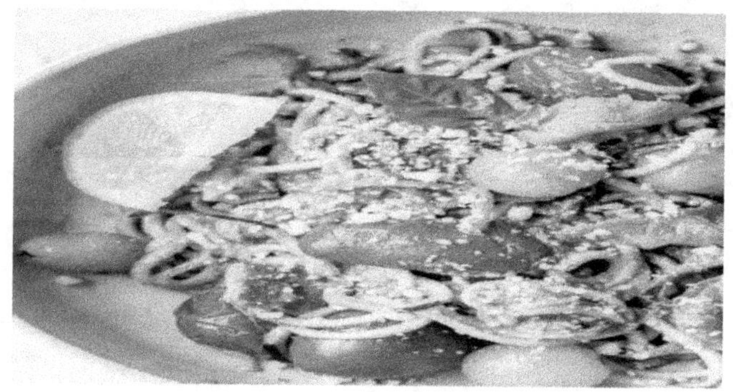

3. Title: Paleo Grilled Chicken and Asparagus

Description: A paleo-friendly dinner featuring grilled chicken breasts and fresh asparagus.

Serving Size: 4 servings

Prep Time: 10 minutes

Cooking Time: 15 minutes

Ingredients:

- 4 boneless, skinless chicken breasts
- 1 pound asparagus spears
- 2 tablespoons olive oil

- 2 cloves garlic, minced
- 1 teaspoon dried oregano
- 1 teaspoon smoked paprika
- Salt and pepper to taste
- Lemon wedges for garnish

Instructions:

1. Season the chicken breasts with olive oil, minced garlic, dried oregano, smoked paprika, salt, and pepper.
2. Preheat the grill to medium-high heat.
3. Grill the chicken breasts for about 6-8 minutes on each side, or until they are cooked through.
4. In a separate grill basket or foil packet, grill asparagus spears until they are tender and slightly charred.
5. Serve your paleo grilled chicken with asparagus, garnished with lemon wedges.

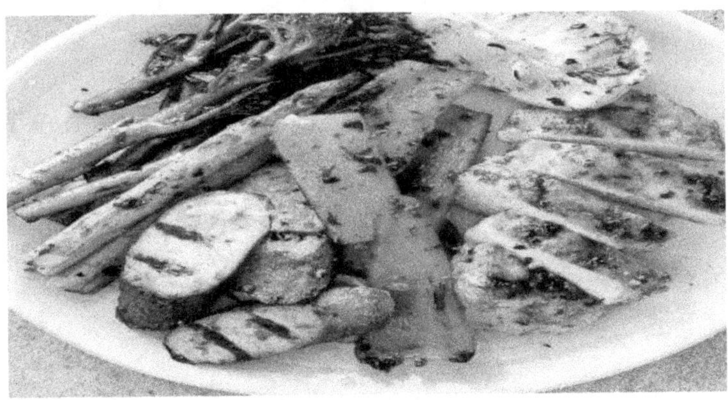

4. Title: Gluten-Free Quinoa Stuffed Bell Peppers

Description: A gluten-free dinner option featuring quinoa and black bean-stuffed bell peppers.

Serving Size: 4 servings

Prep Time: 20 minutes

Cooking Time: 45 minutes

Ingredients:

- 4 bell peppers, any color
- 1 cup cooked quinoa
- 1 can (15 oz) black beans, drained and rinsed
- 1 cup corn kernels (fresh or frozen, thawed)
- 1/4 cup red onion, finely chopped
- 1/4 cup fresh cilantro, chopped
- 1 teaspoon cumin
- Salt and pepper to taste
- 1 cup tomato sauce

Instructions:

1. Preheat the oven to 375°F (190°C).
2. Cut the tops off the bell peppers and remove the seeds.
3. In a large bowl, combine cooked quinoa, black beans, corn, red onion, cilantro, cumin, salt, and pepper.
4. Stuff the bell peppers with the quinoa and black bean mixture.
5. Place the stuffed peppers in a baking dish and pour tomato sauce over them.
6. Cover with foil and bake for about 35-40 minutes or until peppers are tender.
7. Serve your gluten-free quinoa stuffed bell peppers.

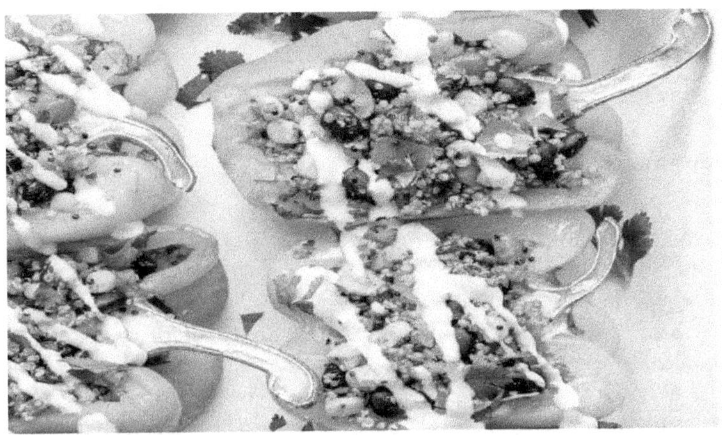

5. Title: Keto-Friendly Grilled Salmon with Avocado Salsa

Description: A keto-friendly dinner featuring grilled salmon and a refreshing avocado salsa.

Serving Size: 4 servings

Prep Time: 15 minutes

Cooking Time: 15 minutes

Ingredients:

- 4 salmon fillets
- 2 tablespoons olive oil
- 1 teaspoon paprika
- 1 teaspoon garlic powder
- Salt and pepper to taste

For the Avocado Salsa:

- 2 avocados, diced
- 1/2 red onion, finely chopped

- 1/4 cup fresh cilantro, chopped
- Juice of 1 lime
- Salt and pepper to taste

Instructions:

1. Season the salmon fillets with olive oil, paprika, garlic powder, salt, and pepper.
2. Preheat the grill to medium-high heat.
3. Grill the salmon for about 4-5 minutes on each side or until it is cooked to your liking.
4. In a bowl, combine diced avocados, chopped red onion, fresh cilantro, lime juice, salt, and pepper to make the salsa.
5. Serve the grilled salmon topped with the avocado salsa.

These dietary-specific dinner options cater to a range of preferences, whether you're following a vegan, low-carb,

These special dinner recipes are perfect for gatherings and celebrations, showcasing a range of flavors and ingredients that are sure to impress your guests and elevate any occasion.

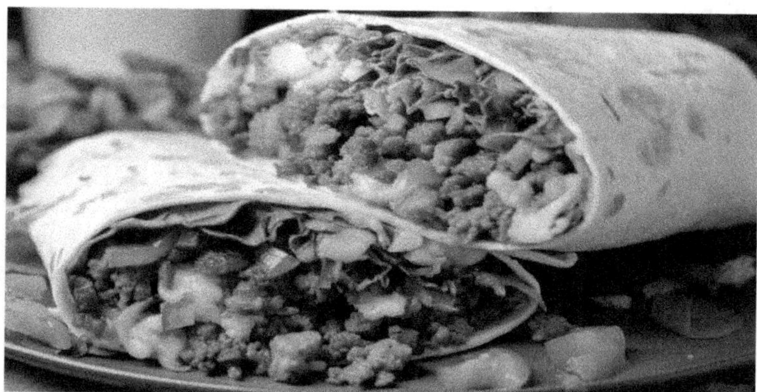

Chapter Six

Nourishing Snacks and Side Dishes

Through this gastronomic exploration, we explore the pleasant realm of "Nourishing Snacks and Side Dishes." Here, we delve into the artistry of creating appetizers and snacks that satisfy your palate and supply the nourishment required for long-lasting vitality. These side dishes are meant to go well with your main courses, enhancing each bite with a different layer of taste and texture.

Delicious and Nutrient-Rich Snacks for Sustained Energy

These delicious and nutrient-rich snacks are perfect for sustaining your energy throughout the day. Whether you prefer the crunch of roasted chickpeas, the creaminess of a yogurt parfait, or the simplicity of apple slices with peanut butter, these snacks offer both taste and nourishment.

Snacking may provide prolonged energy and nutrients, serving as more than simply a temporary solution to hunger. We present a selection of tasty and nutrient-dense snacks in this area. No matter where your day takes you, these snacks will keep you energized and full. They range from protein-rich selections to bite-sized treats that will boost your energy.

1. **Nutty Energy Bites**

Description: These little powerhouses are packed with nuts, seeds, and dried fruits, offering a quick energy boost when you need it.

Serving Size: 12 bites

Prep Time: 15 minutes

Ingredients:

* 1 cup rolled oats
* 1/2 cup almond butter
* 1/4 cup honey
* 1/4 cup chia seeds
* 1/4 cup chopped dried apricots
* 1/4 cup chopped nuts (e.g., almonds, walnuts)
* 1/4 cup mini chocolate chips (optional)
* 1 teaspoon vanilla extract
* A pinch of salt

Instructions:

1. In a large bowl, combine rolled oats, almond butter, honey, chia seeds, chopped dried apricots, chopped nuts, chocolate chips (if using), vanilla extract, and a pinch of salt.
2. Mix well until all ingredients are evenly distributed.
3. Refrigerate the mixture for about 15 minutes to make it easier to handle.
4. Roll the mixture into small bites and place them on a baking sheet.
5. Refrigerate until firm, and then transfer to an airtight container.
6. Grab a nutty energy bite whenever you need a quick energy pick-me-up.

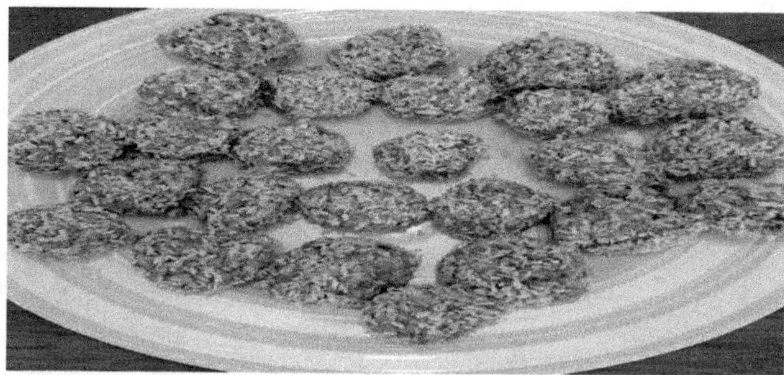

2. **Greek Yogurt Parfait**

Description: A creamy and fruity parfait that's rich in protein, probiotics, and vitamins.

Serving Size: 1 parfait

Prep Time: 5 minutes

Ingredients:

- 1 cup Greek yogurt
- 1/2 cup fresh mixed berries (e.g., strawberries, blueberries, raspberries)
- 2 tablespoons honey
- 1/4 cup granola
- A sprinkle of cinnamon (optional)

Instructions:

1. In a glass or jar, start with a layer of Greek yogurt.
2. Add a layer of fresh mixed berries.
3. Drizzle honey over the berries.
4. Sprinkle granola on top.
5. Repeat the layers if desired.
6. Finish with a sprinkle of cinnamon, if using.
7. Enjoy your creamy Greek yogurt parfait as a wholesome snack.

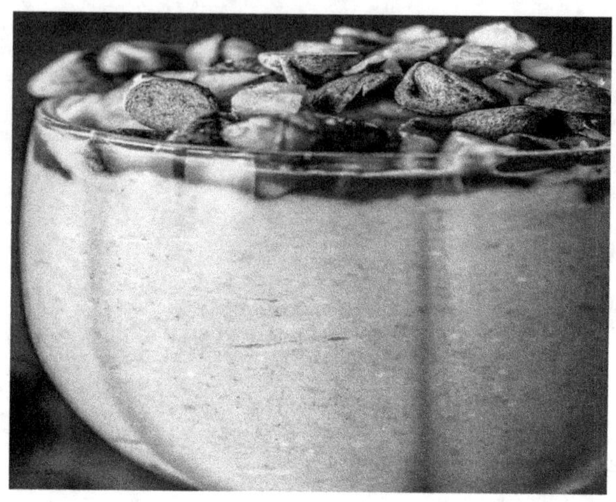

3. **Title: Spiced Roasted Chickpeas**

Description: These crunchy chickpeas are seasoned with spices, making them a satisfying and protein-packed snack.

Serving Size: 2 servings

Prep Time: 5 minutes

Cooking Time: 25 minutes

Ingredients:

- 1 can (15 oz) chickpeas, drained and rinsed
- 2 tablespoons olive oil
- 1 teaspoon cumin
- 1/2 teaspoon paprika
- 1/2 teaspoon garlic powder
- Salt and pepper to taste

Instructions:

1. Preheat the oven to 400°F (200°C).
2. In a bowl, toss chickpeas with olive oil, cumin, paprika, garlic powder, salt, and pepper.
3. Spread the chickpeas on a baking sheet in a single layer.
4. Roast for about 20-25 minutes, or until they are crispy and golden.
5. Let them cool before enjoying your spiced roasted chickpeas.

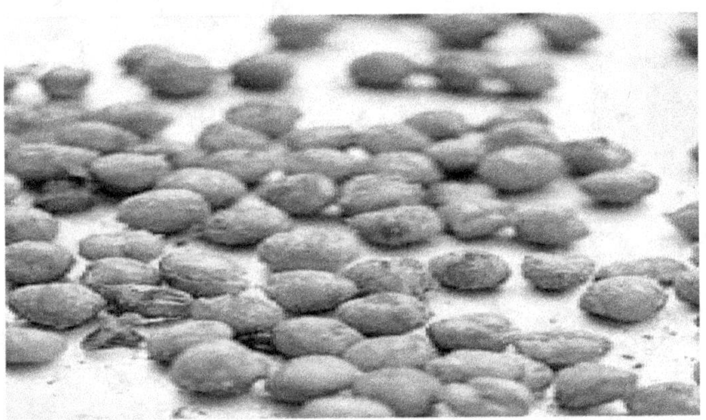

4. Title: Apple and Peanut Butter Slices

Description: A classic combo of apple slices and peanut butter for a satisfying and nutritious snack.

Serving Size: 2 servings

Prep Time: 5 minutes

Ingredients:

- 2 apples, sliced
- 4 tablespoons peanut butter
- Honey and cinnamon for drizzling (optional)

Instructions:

1. Slice the apples.
2. Serve them with a side of peanut butter for dipping.
3. Drizzle with honey and sprinkle cinnamon for added flavor, if desired.
4. Enjoy this simple yet nutritious snack.

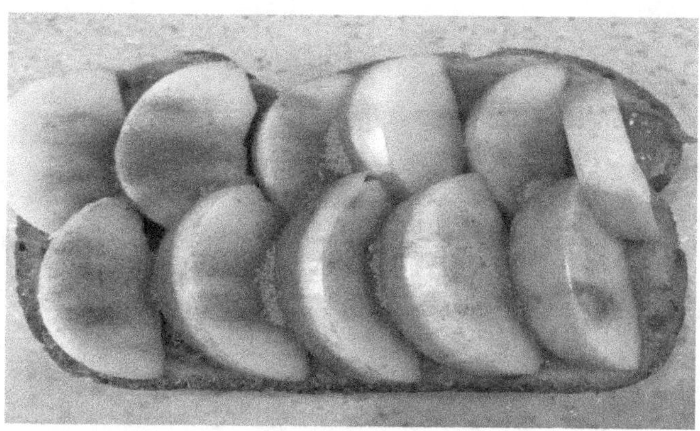

5. Title: Quinoa and Edamame Salad

Description: A protein-packed salad with quinoa and edamame that's perfect for on-the-go energy.

Serving Size: 2 servings

Prep Time: 10 minutes

Ingredients:

- 1 cup cooked quinoa

- 1 cup shelled edamame (steamed or boiled)
- 1/2 cup cherry tomatoes, halved
- 1/4 cup red onion, finely chopped
- 1/4 cup fresh parsley, chopped
- 2 tablespoons lemon juice
- 2 tablespoons olive oil
- Salt and pepper to taste

Instructions:

1. In a large bowl, combine cooked quinoa, shelled edamame, cherry tomatoes, red onion, and fresh parsley.
2. In a separate bowl, whisk together lemon juice, olive oil, salt, and pepper to make the dressing.
3. Drizzle the dressing over the quinoa and edamame salad and toss to combine.
4. Pack it in a container for a nutrient-rich snack on the go.

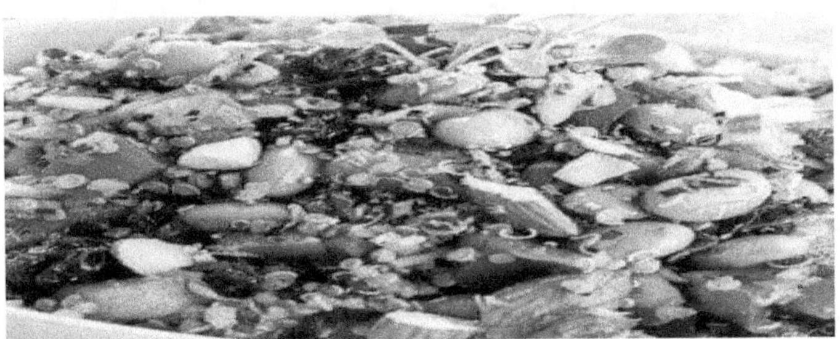

Appetizers and Sides That Complement Your Main Meals

We have an amazing assortment of appetizers and side dishes to complement any meal, and they will make your dining experience even more enjoyable. These recipes are meant to go well with your main courses, whether you're having a dinner party or just having a nice family supper. These appetizers and sides, which range from light salads to filling grains, are the ideal complement to your culinary masterpieces.

1. Caprese Salad Skewers

Description: A delightful and colorful appetizer that combines the freshness of tomatoes, mozzarella, and basil, all on a convenient skewer.

Serving Size: 4 servings

Prep Time: 15 minutes

Ingredients:

- 16 cherry tomatoes
- 16 fresh mozzarella balls
- 16 fresh basil leaves
- 2 tablespoons extra-virgin olive oil
- Balsamic glaze for drizzling
- Salt and pepper to taste

Instructions:

1. Thread a cherry tomato, a mozzarella ball, and a basil leaf onto each skewer.
2. Arrange the skewers on a serving platter.
3. Drizzle with extra-virgin olive oil and balsamic glaze.
4. Season with salt and pepper.
5. Serve these Caprese salad skewers for a burst of flavor and freshness.

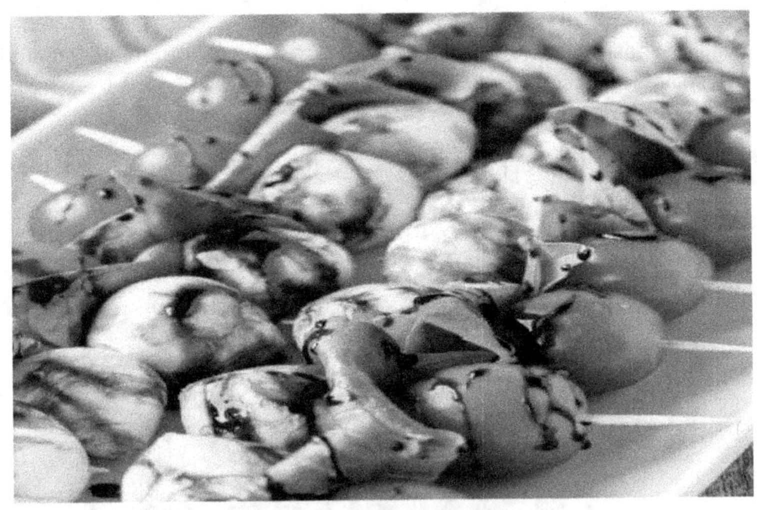

2. Title: Garlic Parmesan Roasted Asparagus

Description: A flavorful side dish featuring roasted asparagus with a garlicky Parmesan crust.

Serving Size: 4 servings

Prep Time: 10 minutes

Cooking Time: 15 minutes

Ingredients:

- 1 bunch asparagus spears, trimmed
- 2 tablespoons olive oil
- 2 cloves garlic, minced
- 1/4 cup grated Parmesan cheese
- Salt and pepper to taste
- Lemon wedges for garnish

Instructions:

1. Preheat the oven to 400°F (200°C).
2. Place asparagus on a baking sheet. Drizzle with olive oil and sprinkle minced garlic, Parmesan cheese, salt, and pepper.
3. Toss to coat the asparagus evenly.
4. Roast for about 12-15 minutes, or until the asparagus is tender and the Parmesan is golden.
5. Garnish with lemon wedges and serve your garlic Parmesan roasted asparagus.

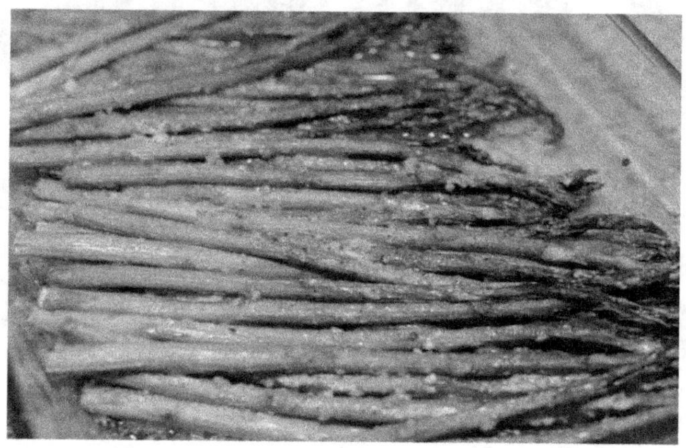

3. Title: Quinoa and Black Bean Salad

Description: A colorful and protein-packed salad with quinoa, black beans, and a zesty lime dressing.

Serving Size: 4 servings

Prep Time: 15 minutes

Ingredients:

- 1 cup cooked quinoa
- 1 can (15 oz) black beans, drained and rinsed

- 1 cup corn kernels (fresh or frozen, thawed)
- 1/4 cup red onion, finely chopped
- 1/4 cup fresh cilantro, chopped
- Juice of 2 limes
- 2 tablespoons olive oil
- Salt and pepper to taste
- Avocado slices for garnish

Instructions:

1. In a large bowl, combine cooked quinoa, black beans, corn, red onion, and fresh cilantro.
2. In a separate bowl, whisk together the lime juice, olive oil, salt, and pepper to make the dressing.
3. Drizzle the dressing over the quinoa and black bean salad and toss to combine.
4. Garnish with avocado slices.
5. Serve this vibrant quinoa and black bean salad as a side dish.

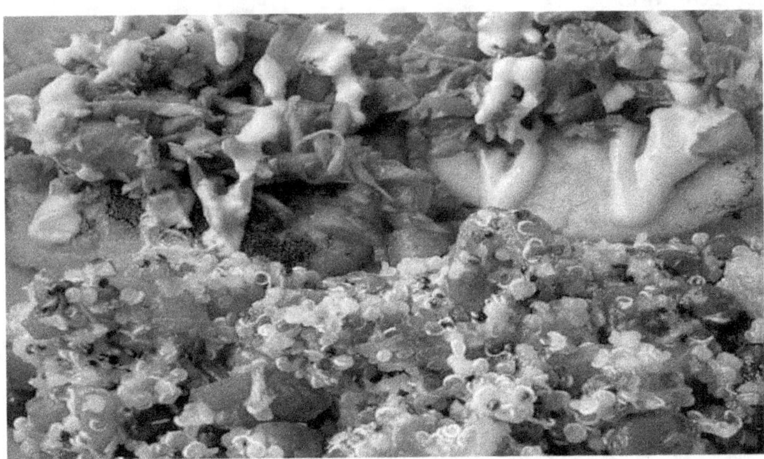

4. Roasted Sweet Potato Fries

Description: Crispy and seasoned sweet potato fries that are the perfect side dish for a variety of main courses.

Serving Size: 4 servings

Prep Time: 10 minutes

Cooking Time: 30 minutes

Ingredients:

- 2 large sweet potatoes, cut into fries
- 2 tablespoons olive oil
- 1 teaspoon paprika
- 1/2 teaspoon garlic powder
- 1/2 teaspoon cumin
- Salt and pepper to taste

Instructions:

1. Preheat the oven to 425°F (220°C).
2. In a large bowl, toss sweet potato fries with olive oil, paprika, garlic powder, cumin, salt, and pepper.
3. Spread the fries on a baking sheet in a single layer.
4. Roast for about 25-30 minutes, or until they are crispy and golden.
5. Serve your roasted sweet potato fries as a tasty side.

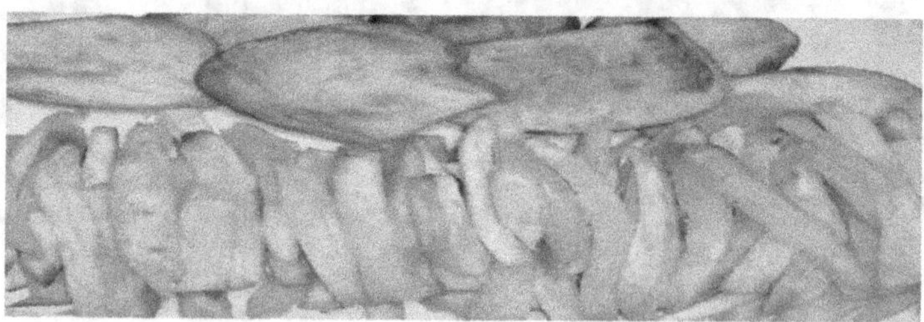

5. Tabbouleh Salad

Description: A refreshing and herby Middle Eastern salad featuring bulgur, tomatoes, cucumbers, and fresh parsley.

Serving Size: 4 servings

Prep Time: 15 minutes

Ingredients:

- 1 cup bulgur wheat
- 1 1/2 cups boiling water
- 2 tomatoes, diced
- 1 cucumber, diced
- 1/2 cup fresh parsley, chopped
- 1/4 cup fresh mint leaves, chopped
- Juice of 2 lemons
- 1/4 cup extra-virgin olive oil
- Salt and pepper to taste

Instructions:

1. Place bulgur wheat in a bowl and pour boiling water over it. Cover and let it sit for about 15 minutes, or until it's tender.
2. Fluff the cooked bulgur with a fork and let it cool.
3. In a large bowl, combine bulgur, diced tomatoes, diced cucumber, fresh parsley, and fresh mint.
4. In a separate bowl, whisk together lemon juice, extra-virgin olive oil, salt, and pepper to make the dressing.
5. Drizzle the dressing over the tabbouleh salad and toss to combine.
6. Serve this refreshing tabbouleh salad as a side dish.

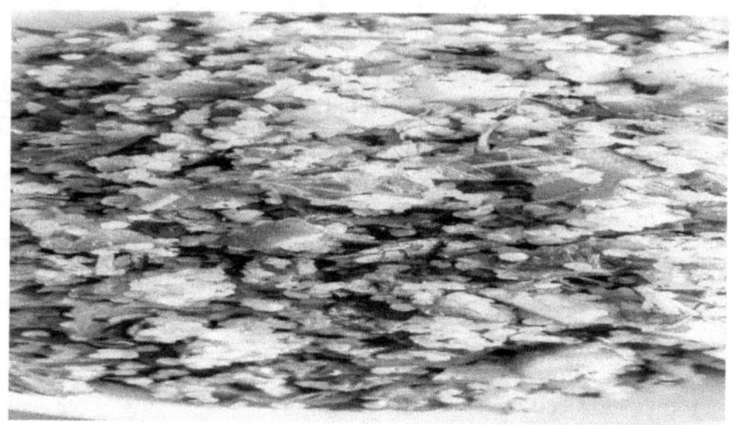

These appetizers and side dishes are a delightful addition to your main meals, offering a variety of flavors and textures to enhance your dining experience. Whether it's the classic Caprese salad skewers or the zesty quinoa and black bean salad, each recipe is designed to complement your main courses with flair and taste.

Snack and Side Dish Alternatives for Various Diets

We are aware that there are many different dietary choices and limitations. For this reason, we've selected a variety of side dish and snack options to accommodate various dietary requirements. There are alternatives to suit your nutritional preferences, be it vegan, gluten-free, keto, or any other specialized diet. No one, regardless of dietary requirements, has to give up taste or fun thanks to these recipes.

1. Vegan Cauliflower Buffalo Bites

Description: A vegan take on buffalo wings, these cauliflower bites are spicy and flavorful, perfect for a plant-based diet.

Serving Size: 4 servings

Prep Time: 15 minutes

Cooking Time: 25 minutes

Ingredients:

- 1 head cauliflower, cut into florets
- 1/2 cup flour (use a gluten-free flour if needed)
- 1/2 cup water
- 1 teaspoon garlic powder
- 1/2 cup hot sauce (check for vegan options)
- 2 tablespoons vegan butter
- Salt and pepper to taste

Instructions:

1. Preheat the oven to 450°F (230°C).
2. In a bowl, whisk together flour, water, garlic powder, salt, and pepper to make a batter.
3. Dip cauliflower florets into the batter, ensuring they are well-coated.
4. Place the battered florets on a baking sheet and bake for about 20 minutes, or until they're crispy.
5. In a saucepan, melt vegan butter and hot sauce, and toss the baked cauliflower in the sauce.
6. Return to the oven for an additional 5 minutes.
7. Serve your vegan cauliflower buffalo bites with a dairy-free dip of your choice.

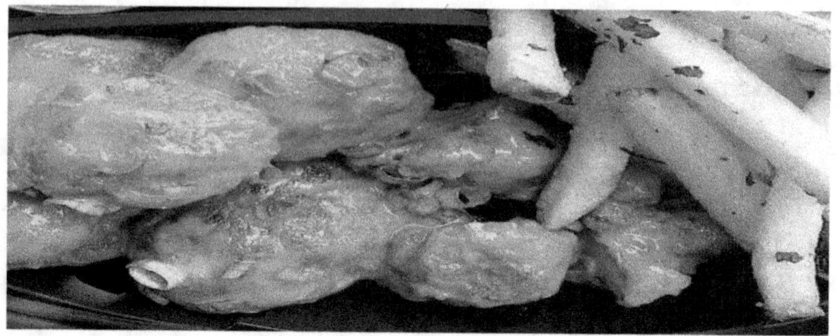

2. Title: Low-Carb Cucumber Sushi Rolls

Description: A low-carb alternative to sushi using cucumber as a wrapper, perfect for a keto or low-carb diet.

Serving Size: 2 servings

Prep Time: 15 minutes

Ingredients:

- 2 large cucumbers
- 1 cup crab or imitation crab meat (check for low-carb options)
- 1/2 avocado, sliced
- 1/4 cup cream cheese (use a low-carb or dairy-free option if needed)
- Soy sauce or coconut aminos for dipping

Instructions:

1. Slice the cucumbers lengthwise into thin strips using a mandoline or a vegetable peeler.
2. Lay out a cucumber strip and place a small amount of crab or imitation crab meat, avocado, and a small amount of cream cheese at one end.

3. Roll the cucumber strip tightly, similar to a sushi roll.
4. Repeat for the remaining cucumber strips.
5. Slice the rolls into bite-sized pieces.
6. Serve your low-carb cucumber sushi rolls with soy sauce or coconut aminos for dipping.

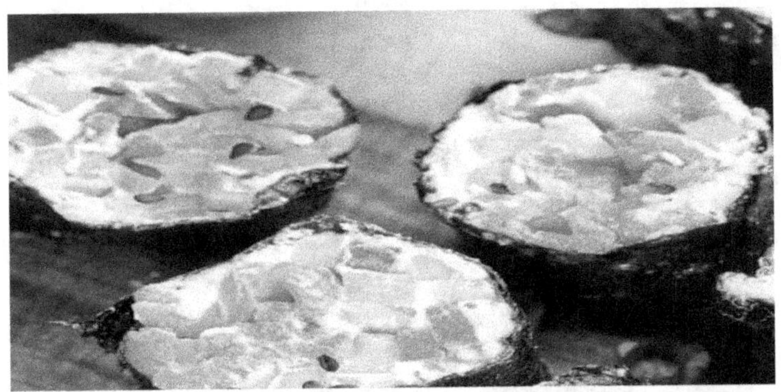

3. Gluten-Free Quinoa and Black Bean Stuffed Peppers

Description: These stuffed peppers are gluten-free and packed with quinoa and black beans, suitable for those with gluten sensitivities.

Serving Size: 4 servings

Prep Time: 15 minutes

Cooking Time: 45 minutes

Ingredients:

- 4 bell peppers, any color
- 1 cup cooked quinoa
- 1 can (15 oz) black beans, drained and rinsed
- 1 cup corn kernels (fresh or frozen, thawed)
- 1/4 cup red onion, finely chopped
- 1/4 cup fresh cilantro, chopped
- 1 teaspoon cumin

- Salt and pepper to taste
- 1 cup tomato sauce

Instructions:

1. Preheat the oven to 375°F (190°C).
2. Cut the tops off the bell peppers and remove the seeds.
3. In a large bowl, combine cooked quinoa, black beans, corn, red onion, cilantro, cumin, salt, and pepper.
4. Stuff the bell peppers with the quinoa and black bean mixture.
5. Place the stuffed peppers in a baking dish and pour tomato sauce over them.
6. Cover with foil and bake for about 35-40 minutes, or until peppers are tender.
7. Serve your gluten-free quinoa and black bean stuffed peppers.

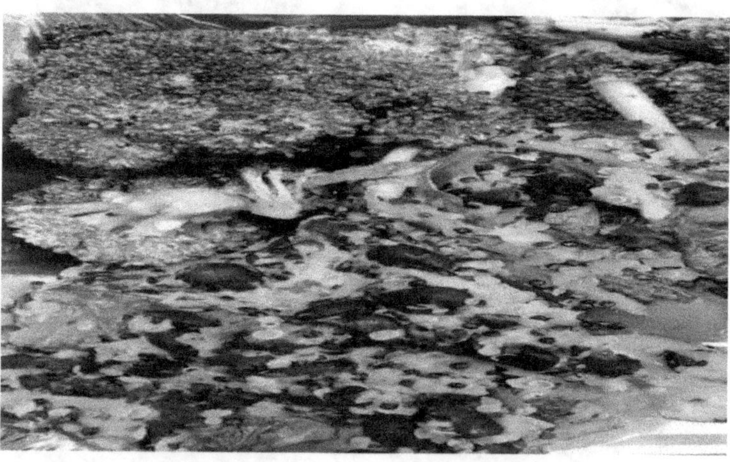

4. Keto-Friendly Zucchini Noodles with Pesto

Description: A keto-friendly alternative to pasta using zucchini noodles and a flavorful pesto sauce.

Serving Size: 2 servings

Prep Time: 15 minutes

Ingredients:

- 2 large zucchinis
- 1 cup fresh basil leaves
- 1/4 cup pine nuts
- 2 cloves garlic
- 1/4 cup nutritional yeast (for a cheesy flavor)
- 1/4 cup olive oil
- Juice of 1 lemon
- Salt and pepper to taste

Instructions:

1. Use a spiralizer to create zucchini noodles from the zucchinis.
2. In a food processor, combine fresh basil, pine nuts, garlic, nutritional yeast, olive oil, lemon juice, salt, and pepper. Blend into a pesto sauce.
3. Toss the zucchini noodles with the pesto sauce until well coated.
4. Serve your keto-friendly zucchini noodles with pesto.

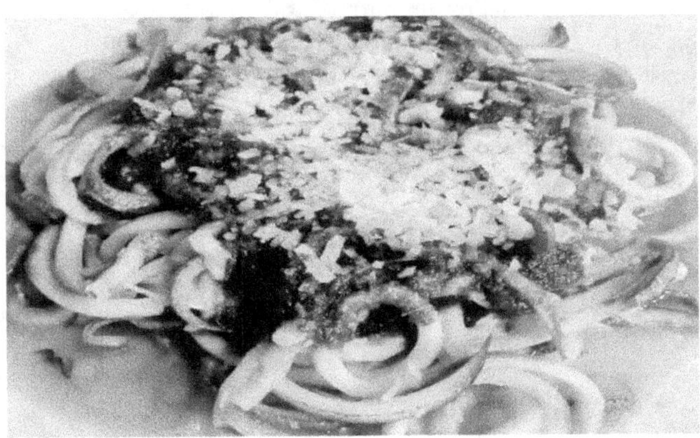

5. Paleo Roasted Butternut Squash

Description: A paleo-friendly side dish featuring roasted butternut squash with a blend of spices and herbs.

Serving Size: 4 servings

Prep Time: 10 minutes

Cooking Time: 25 minutes

Ingredients:

- 1 butternut squash, peeled, seeded, and diced
- 2 tablespoons coconut oil
- 1 teaspoon ground cinnamon
- 1/2 teaspoon ground nutmeg
- Salt and pepper to taste

Instructions:

1. Preheat the oven to 400°F (200°C).
2. In a large bowl, toss the diced butternut squash with coconut oil, ground cinnamon, ground nutmeg, salt, and pepper.
3. Spread the seasoned squash on a baking sheet.
4. Roast for about 20-25 minutes, or until the squash is tender and slightly caramelized.
5. Serve your paleo roasted butternut squash as a delicious and diet-friendly side dish.

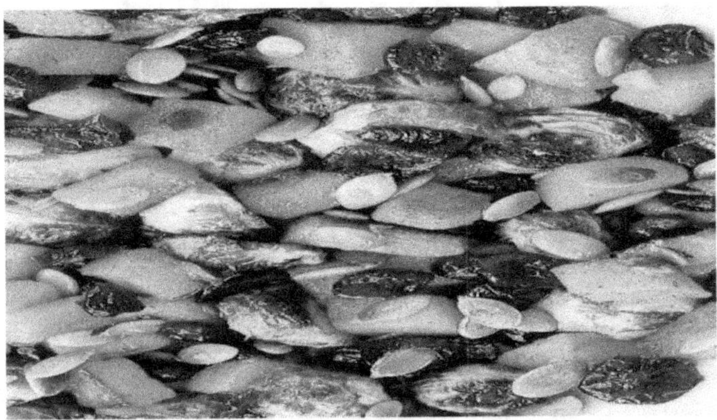

These snack and side dish alternatives are designed to accommodate different dietary preferences, whether you're following a vegan, low-carb, gluten-free, keto, or paleo diet. Enjoy flavorful and satisfying options that align with your dietary choices.

We honor the artistry of nibbling and the importance of thoughtfully prepared side dishes in Chapter 6. Our dishes, which range from delectable snacks to sides that round out your meals, are a testament to the harmonious combination of flavor and nutrition. Discover the gastronomic options and enhance your eating experience with filling appetizers and side dishes that satiate the mind and body.

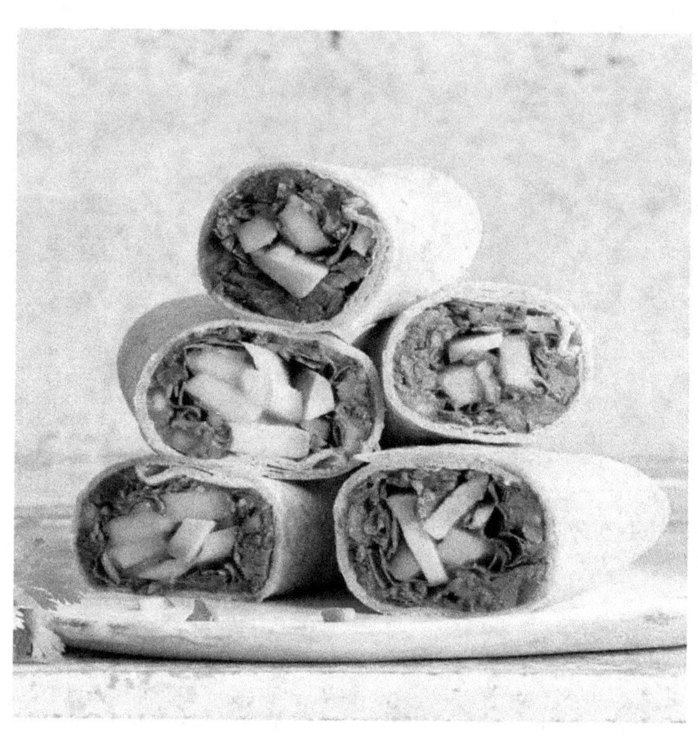

Chapter Seven

Sweet Endings that Defy Aging

Get ready to go on a delicious adventure into the world of "Sweet Endings that Defy Aging." This last chapter delves into the skill of creating sweets that fulfill your sweet taste while also upholding the values of a youthful, healthy way of living. You may have your cake and eat it too, guilt-free, as we provide you with an enticing assortment of decadent and nutritious sweets.

Desserts That Are Both Healthy and Indulgent

Say goodbye to the belief that indulging would negatively impact your health. We provide treats that harmoniously combine health and deliciousness. These desserts, which range from yogurt parfaits with fresh berries on top to velvety avocado chocolate mousse, exhibit the ideal harmony between flavor and nutrition.

1. Creamy Avocado Chocolate Mousse

Description: A rich and creamy chocolate mousse that gets its velvety texture from ripe avocados, making it a guilt-free dessert.

Serving Size: 4 servings

Prep Time: 10 minutes

Ingredients:

- 2 ripe avocados, peeled and pitted
- 1/4 cup unsweetened cocoa powder
- 1/4 cup honey or maple syrup
- 1/4 cup almond milk (or any milk of your choice)
- 1 teaspoon vanilla extract
- A pinch of salt

- Fresh berries for garnish

Instructions:

1. In a food processor, combine ripe avocados, cocoa powder, honey or maple syrup, almond milk, vanilla extract, and a pinch of salt.
2. Blend until the mixture is smooth and creamy.
3. Divide the chocolate mousse into serving glasses or bowls.
4. Refrigerate for at least 30 minutes.
5. Garnish with fresh berries before serving.

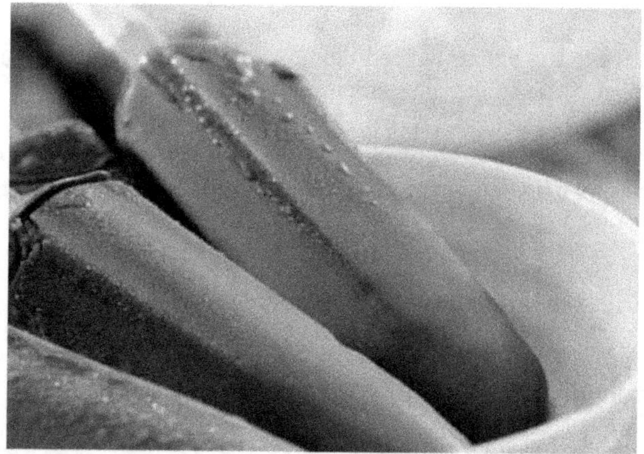

2. Greek Yogurt Parfait with Fresh Berries

Description: A parfait featuring Greek yogurt and a medley of fresh berries, offering a balance of creaminess and natural sweetness.

Serving Size: 2 servings

Prep Time: 5 minutes

Ingredients:

- 1 cup Greek yogurt
- 1/2 cup fresh mixed berries (e.g., strawberries, blueberries, raspberries)
- 2 tablespoons honey or maple syrup
- 1/4 cup granola
- A sprinkle of cinnamon (optional)

Instructions:

1. In a glass or jar, start with a layer of Greek yogurt.
2. Add a layer of fresh mixed berries.
3. Drizzle honey or maple syrup over the berries.
4. Sprinkle granola on top.
5. Repeat the layers if desired.
6. Finish with a sprinkle of cinnamon, if using.
7. Enjoy your creamy Greek yogurt parfait with fresh berries.

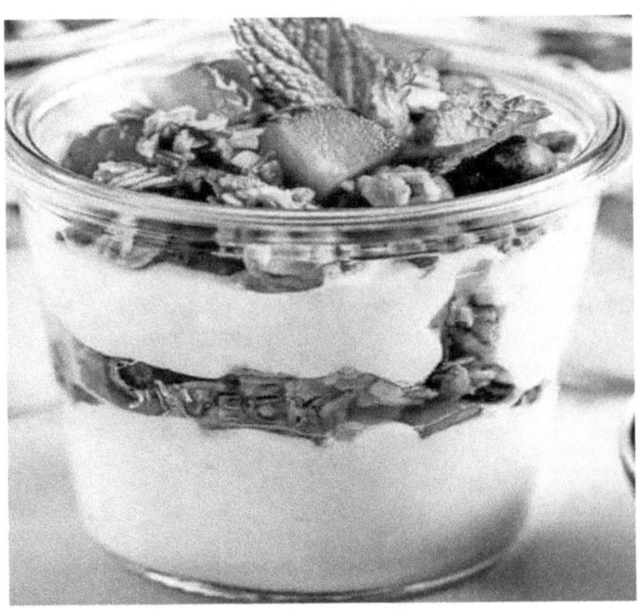

3. Chia Seed Pudding with Coconut and Mango

Description: A tropical-inspired chia seed pudding made with coconut milk and fresh mango, providing a luscious and healthy dessert.

Serving Size: 2 servings

Prep Time: 5 minutes

Ingredients:

- 1/4 cup chia seeds
- 1 cup coconut milk
- 1 tablespoon honey or maple syrup
- 1/2 teaspoon vanilla extract
- 1 ripe mango, diced
- Unsweetened shredded coconut for garnish

Instructions:

1. In a bowl, combine chia seeds, coconut milk, honey or maple syrup, and vanilla extract.
2. Stir well and let it sit for 10 minutes, then stir again to avoid clumping.
3. Cover the bowl and refrigerate for at least 4 hours or overnight.
4. To serve, layer the chia seed pudding with diced mango in serving glasses.
5. Garnish with unsweetened shredded coconut.
6. Enjoy your tropical chia seed pudding with coconut and mango.

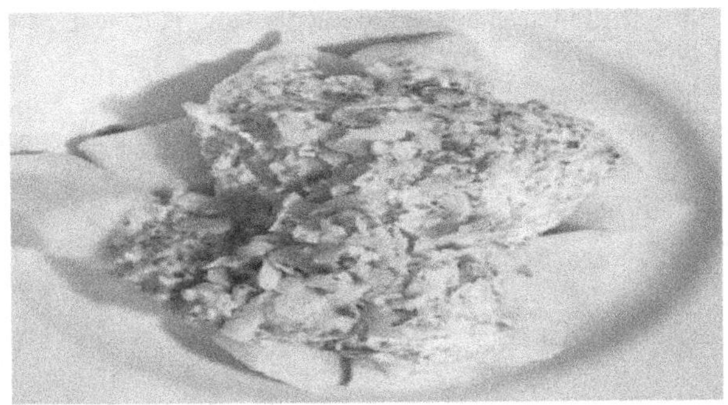

4. Baked Apples with Cinnamon and Walnuts

Description: Warm and tender baked apples filled with a mixture of cinnamon, walnuts, and a hint of sweetness.

Serving Size: 4 servings

Prep Time: 10 minutes

Cooking Time: 35 minutes

Ingredients:

- 4 apples, cored and halved
- 1/4 cup chopped walnuts
- 2 tablespoons honey or maple syrup
- 1 teaspoon ground cinnamon
- 1/4 cup water

Instructions:

1. Preheat the oven to 350°F (175°C).
2. In a bowl, combine chopped walnuts, honey or maple syrup, and ground cinnamon.
3. Fill the apple halves with the walnut mixture.

4. Place the stuffed apples in a baking dish and pour water into the dish.
5. Cover with foil and bake for about 25 minutes.
6. Remove the foil and bake for an additional 10 minutes, or until the apples are tender.
7. Serve your baked apples with cinnamon and walnuts while they're warm.

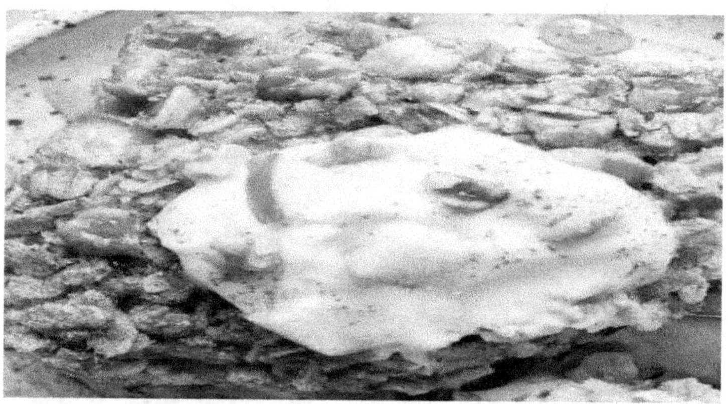

5. Frozen Banana and Peanut Butter Bites

Description: Frozen banana slices with a dollop of peanut butter, offering a delightful and satisfying frozen treat.

Serving Size: 4 servings

Prep Time: 15 minutes

Freezing Time: 2 hours

Ingredients:

- 2 ripe bananas, peeled and sliced into rounds
- 1/4 cup peanut butter
- 1/4 cup dark chocolate chips (optional)
- Chopped nuts (e.g., almonds, walnuts) for garnish (optional)

Instructions:

1. Spread a small amount of peanut butter on one banana slice and top it with another to create a banana "sandwich."
2. Continue making banana "sandwiches" until all slices are used.
3. Place the banana and peanut butter bites on a baking sheet lined with parchment paper.
4. If desired, melt dark chocolate chips and drizzle it over

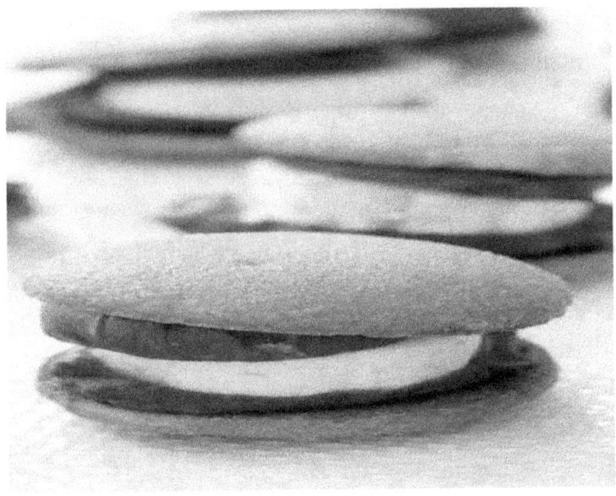

Options for Sugar-Free and Allergy-Friendly Desserts

We are aware that everyone has different dietary needs and sensitivities, and this variety is reflected in our selection of desserts. You may discover a variety of delicious snacks that meet your individual requirements, whether you're looking for sugar-free goodies or desserts that accept common allergies like gluten or nuts.

1. Raw Vegan Brownies

Description: These fudgy brownies are made with wholesome ingredients and are free of refined sugar, gluten, and dairy. They're perfect for satisfying your sweet tooth without any guilt.

Serving Size: 8
Prep Time: 15 minutes
Cooking Time: None

Ingredients:
- 1 cup raw walnuts
- 1 cup pitted dates
- 1/3 cup unsweetened cocoa powder
- 1/4 cup almond flour
- 1/4 tsp sea salt

Instructions:
1. In a food processor, blend the walnuts until they're finely ground.
2. Add the dates, cocoa powder, almond flour, and sea salt to the food processor.
3. Blend until the mixture forms a sticky dough.
4. Press the dough into an 8x8 inch baking dish lined with parchment paper.
5. Chill in the refrigerator for at least 30 minutes before slicing and serving.

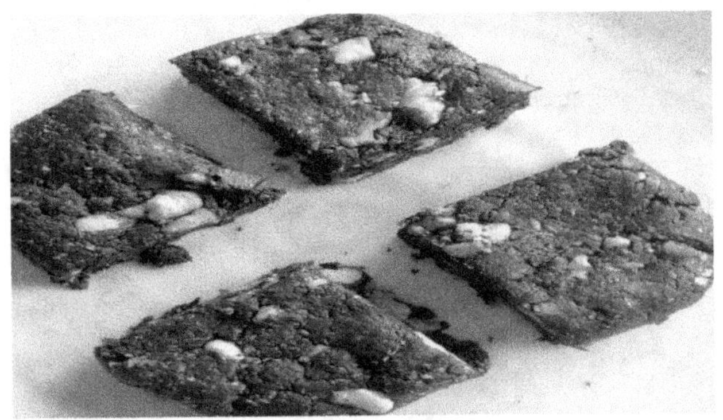

2. Coconut Flour Banana Bread

Description: This moist and flavorful banana bread is made with coconut flour and is free of gluten and refined sugar. It's perfect for breakfast or as a snack.

Serving Size: 8
Prep Time: 10 minutes
Cooking Time: 45 minutes

Ingredients:
- 3 ripe bananas, mashed
- 4 eggs
- 1/4 cup coconut oil, melted
- 1/4 cup honey
- 1 tsp vanilla extract
- 1/2 cup coconut flour
- 1 tsp baking powder
- 1/2 tsp cinnamon

Instructions:
1. Preheat the oven to 350°F (175°C).
2. In a large bowl, whisk together the mashed bananas, eggs, coconut oil, honey, and vanilla extract.

3. In a separate bowl, mix together the coconut flour, baking powder, and cinnamon.

4. Add the dry ingredients to the wet ingredients and mix until well combined.

5. Pour the batter into a greased loaf pan.

6. Bake for 45 minutes or until a toothpick inserted into the center comes out clean.

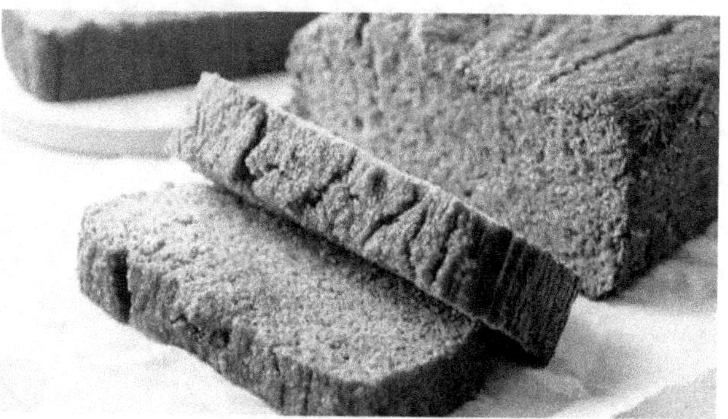

3. Chia Seed Pudding with Berries

Description: This creamy and nutritious pudding is made with chia seeds and almond milk and is sweetened with honey. It's topped with fresh berries for a burst of flavor.

Serving Size: 2
Prep Time: 5 minutes
Cooking Time: None

Ingredients:
- 1/4 cup chia seeds
- 1 cup almond milk
- 2 tbsp honey
- 1 tsp vanilla extract
- Fresh berries for topping

Instructions:

1. In a medium-sized bowl, whisk together the chia seeds, almond milk, honey, and vanilla extract.
2. Let the mixture sit for at least 30 minutes or until it thickens to a pudding-like consistency.
3. Divide the pudding into two bowls and top with fresh berries.

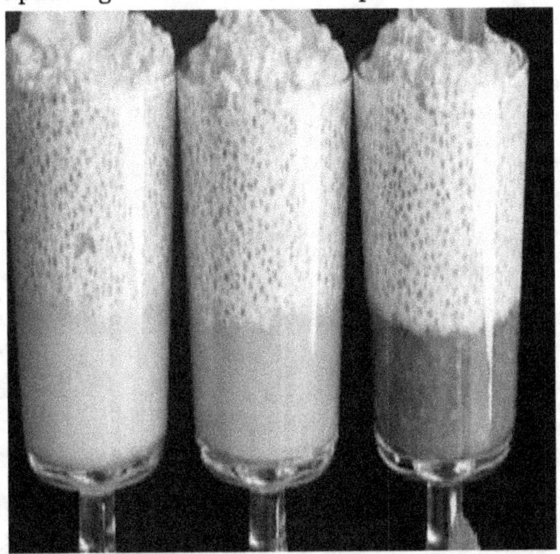

4. No-Bake Peanut Butter Cookies

Description: These cookies are made with just a few simple ingredients and are free of gluten and refined sugar. They're perfect for a quick and easy snack.

Serving Size: 12
Prep Time: 10 minutes
Cooking Time: None

Ingredients:
- 1 cup rolled oats
- 1/2 cup natural peanut butter

- 1/4 cup honey
- 1 tsp vanilla extract

Instructions:
1. In a large bowl, mix together the rolled oats, peanut butter, honey, and vanilla extract.
2. Roll the mixture into balls and flatten them with a fork to create a cookie shape.
3. Chill in the refrigerator for at least 30 minutes before serving.

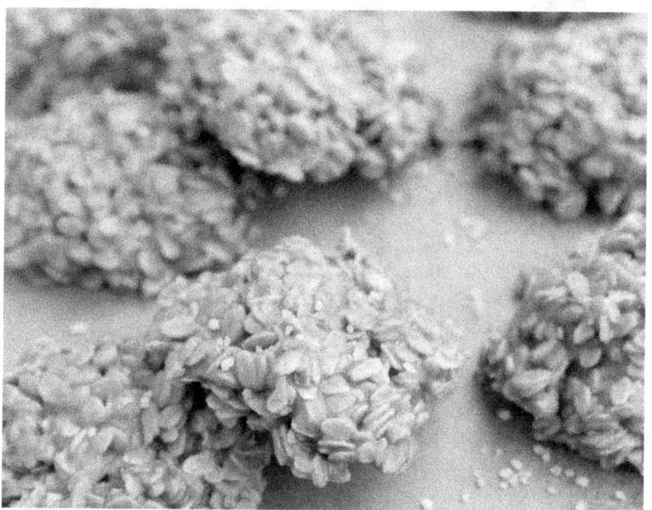

5. Baked Pears with Cinnamon and Almonds

Description: These warm and comforting pears are baked until tender and then topped with a sweet and nutty mixture of cinnamon and almonds.

Serving Size: 4
Prep Time: 10 minutes
Cooking Time: 30 minutes

Ingredients:

- 4 ripe pears
- 2 tbsp honey
- 1 tsp ground cinnamon
- 1/4 cup sliced almonds

Instructions:

1. Preheat the oven to 375°F (190°C).

2. Cut off the top of each pear and scoop out the core.

3. In a small bowl, mix together the honey, cinnamon, and sliced almonds.

4. Stuff each pear with the honey-cinnamon-almond mixture.

5. Place the pears in a baking dish and bake for 30 minutes or until they're tender.

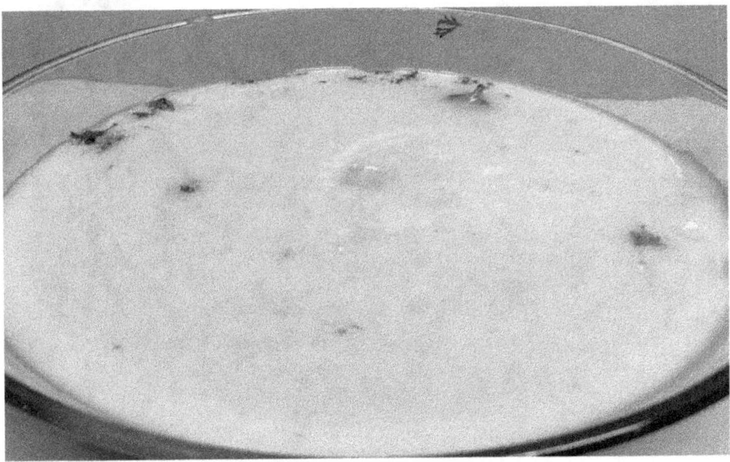

In the realm of "Sweet Endings that Defy Aging," we demonstrate that sweets that keep up with age are not a contradiction. These treats get you closer to that sweet spot where pleasure meets energy with every bite. Come learn about the artistry of creating sweets that will entice your taste buds and keep you looking young and energetic.

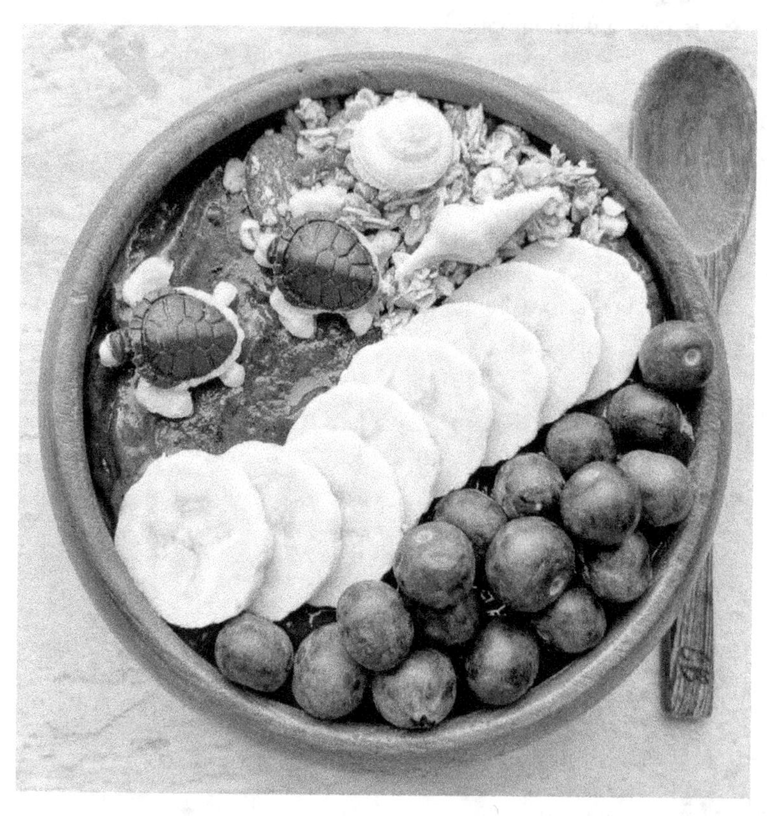

Chapter Eight

Beverages for Radiant Health

Maintaining optimal health requires being hydrated, but did you know that choosing the right beverages may help increase your intake of nutrients and encourage radiant health? We'll look at some nutrient-dense and hydrating beverage options in this chapter that will help you feel renewed and invigorated.

Hydrating and Nutrient-Boosting Beverage Choices

Water is the most important component in the pursuit of radiant health. Find out more options for slaking your thirst besides water. Investigate drinks that provide your body with essential nutrients, such as infused waters, herbal teas, or refreshing coconut water. With each sip, embrace the advantages of age-defying nourishment and stay refreshed.

1. Cucumber Mint Infused Water

Description: A refreshing and low-calorie drink perfect for staying hydrated and promoting healthy skin.

Serving Size: 1 pitcher

Prep Time: 5 minutes

Ingredients:

- 1 cucumber, thinly sliced
- 10-12 fresh mint leaves
- 8 cups of water

Instructions:

1. Add cucumber slices and mint leaves to a pitcher.
2. Pour in 8 cups of water.
3. Refrigerate for at least 1 hour before serving.

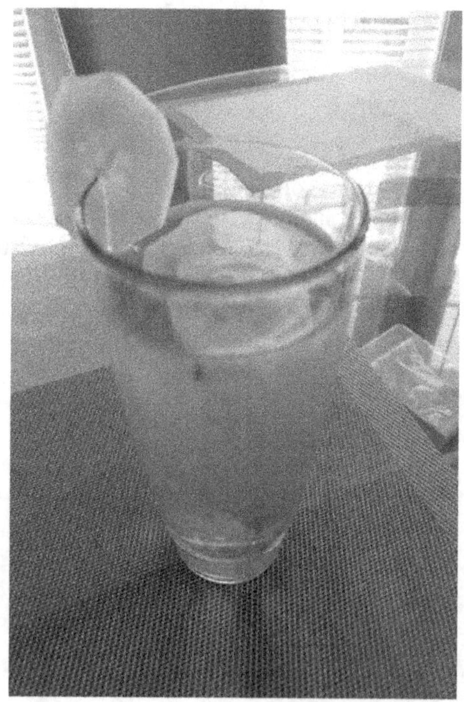

2. Tropical Green Smoothie

Description: A tropical-inspired, vitamin-packed green smoothie for a nutrient boost.

Serving Size: 2 servings

Prep Time: 10 minutes

Cooking Time: 0 minutes

Ingredients:

- 1 cup fresh spinach
- 1/2 cup pineapple chunks
- 1/2 banana
- 1/2 cup coconut milk
- 1/2 cup Greek yogurt
- 1 tablespoon honey (optional)

Instructions:

- Combine all the ingredients in a blender.
- Blend until smooth.
- Serve immediately.

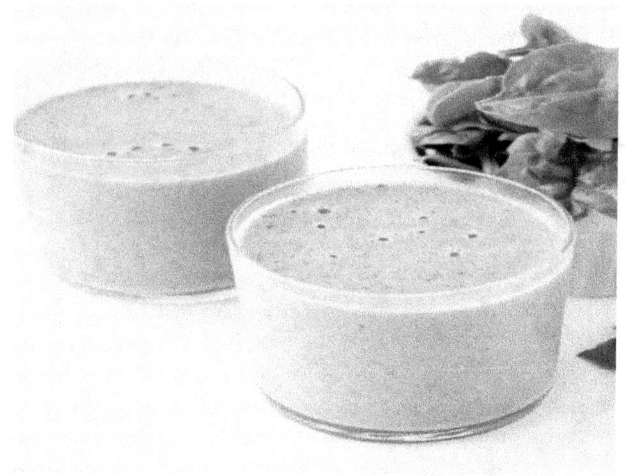

3. **Berry Blast Smoothie**

Description: A delicious and antioxidant-rich smoothie to boost your immune system.

Serving Size: 2 servings

Prep Time: 5 minutes

Cooking Time: 0 minutes

Ingredients:

1. 1 cup mixed berries (strawberries, blueberries, raspberries)
2. 1/2 cup Greek yogurt
3. 1/2 cup almond milk
4. 1 tablespoon honey (optional)

5. Ice cubes

Instructions:

- Place all ingredients in a blender.
- Blend until creamy and smooth.
- Add ice cubes and blend again if you prefer it colder.
- Serve immediately.

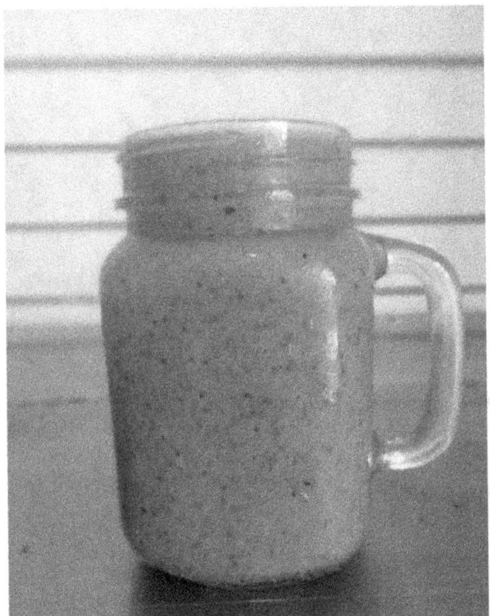

4. **Coconut Water and Pineapple Cooler**

Description: A hydrating and electrolyte-rich drink with a tropical twist.

Serving Size: 1 serving

Prep Time: 5 minutes

Cooking Time: 0 minutes

Ingredients:

- 1 cup coconut water
- 1/2 cup fresh pineapple juice
- Squeeze of lime juice
- Ice cubes

Instructions:

1. In a glass, combine coconut water and pineapple juice.
2. Add a squeeze of lime juice for extra flavor.
3. Add ice cubes, stir, and enjoy!

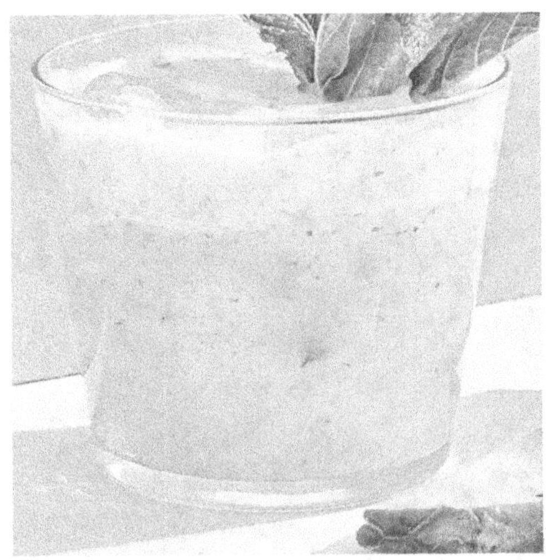

5. **Chia Seed Lemonade**

Description: A citrusy, hydrating drink with the added benefits of chia seeds for fiber and omega-3s.

Serving Size: 2 servings

Prep Time: 5 minutes

Cooking Time: 0 minutes

Ingredients:

1. 2 cups water
2. 2 tablespoons chia seeds
3. Juice of 2 lemons
4. 2-3 tablespoons honey (adjust to taste)

Instructions:

- In a pitcher, combine water, chia seeds, lemon juice, and honey.
- Stir well and let it sit for 10 minutes.
- Stir again and serve with ice.

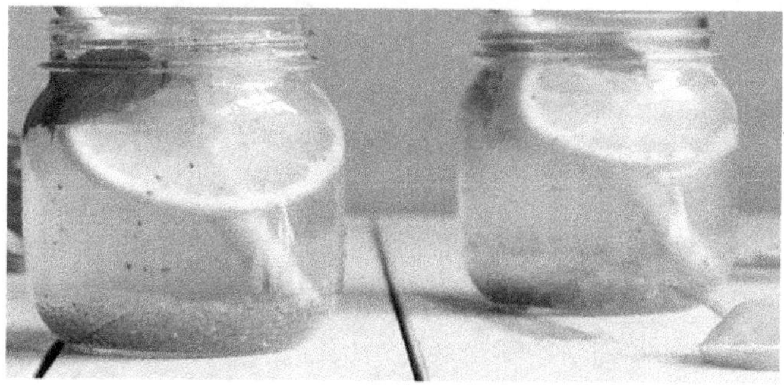

Smoothies, Juices, and Elixirs for Ageless Wellness

Smoothies are a fantastic method to get a lot of nutrients in one tasty beverage that is portable. Your smoothie may be tailored to your dietary requirements and taste preferences. For example, you may include fruits like bananas or berries for fiber and antioxidants, leafy greens like spinach or kale for an increase in vitamins and minerals, and healthy fats like avocado or nut butter for brain function and satiety.

Another method of obtaining a concentrated amount of vitamins and minerals from fruits and vegetables is through juices. To avoid blood sugar spikes, it's crucial to select juices that are high in fiber and low in sugar. If you want the anti-inflammatory properties of herbs, you may also add turmeric or ginger.

Herbal tonics and elixirs are made to help certain health objectives. For instance, an adaptogenic herb elixir for reducing stress would include ashwagandha or rhodiola, while an elixir to improve digestion might include digestive bitters like dandelion or gentian. Elixirs can be poured into other drinks, such as juice or tea, or consumed as shots.

1. Anti-Aging Green Smoothie

Description: Packed with antioxidants and nutrients, this green smoothie helps promote radiant skin and overall vitality.

Serving Size: 2 servings

Prep Time: 10 minutes

Cooking Time: 0 minutes

Ingredients:

- 2 cups fresh spinach
- 1/2 cucumber
- 1/2 avocado
- 1 banana
- 1 cup coconut water
- 1 tablespoon chia seeds

Instructions:

1. Add all ingredients to a blender.
2. Blend until smooth and creamy.
3. Serve immediately.

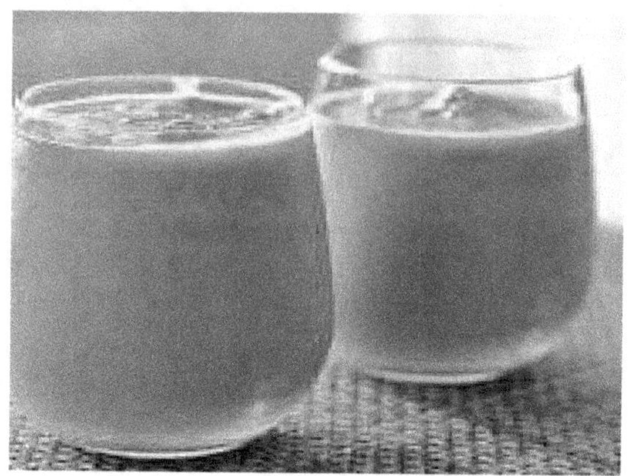

2. **Glowing Skin Carrot and Orange Juice**

Description: This vibrant juice is rich in vitamin C and beta-carotene to support healthy skin and slow down the aging process.

Serving Size: 2 servings

Prep Time: 5 minutes

Cooking Time: 0 minutes

Ingredients:

- 4 large carrots
- 4 oranges, peeled
- 1-inch piece of ginger (optional)

Instructions:

1. Run the carrots, oranges, and ginger (if using) through a juicer.
2. Stir the juice well.
3. Serve immediately over ice.

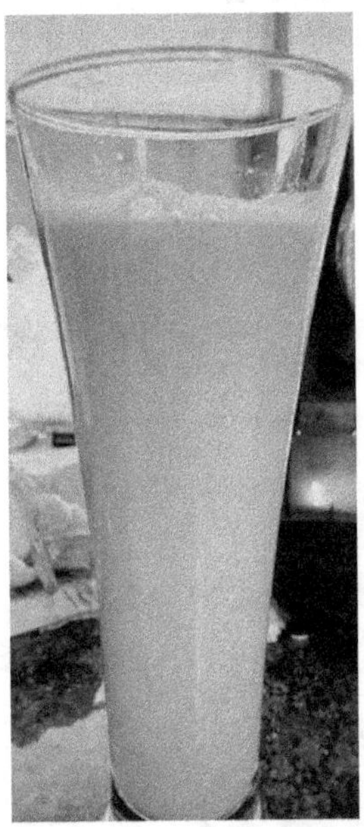

3. Turmeric and Ginger Anti-Inflammatory Elixir

Description: This elixir harnesses the anti-inflammatory properties of turmeric and ginger to support overall well-being.

Serving Size: 2 servings

Prep Time: 5 minutes

Cooking Time: 5 minutes

Ingredients:

- 2 cups water
- 1 teaspoon turmeric powder
- 1 teaspoon fresh grated ginger
- Juice of 1 lemon
- 2 tablespoons honey (adjust to taste)

Instructions:

1. In a saucepan, combine water, turmeric, and ginger.
2. Simmer for 5 minutes, then strain.
3. Stir in lemon juice and honey.
4. Serve warm.

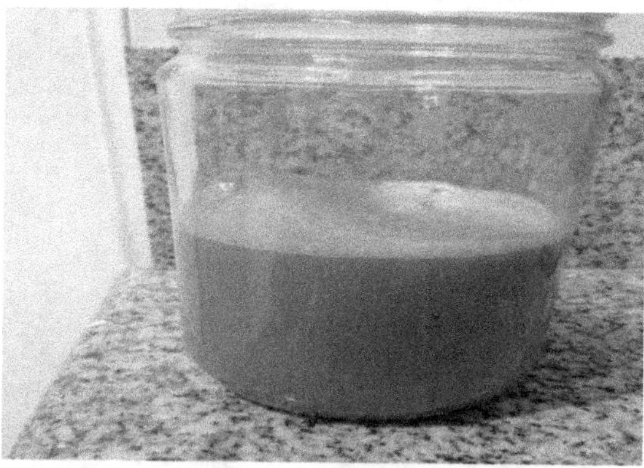

4. Berry-Infused Collagen Smoothie

Description: This collagen-boosting smoothie supports skin elasticity and joint health.

Serving Size: 2 servings

Prep Time: 10 minutes

Cooking Time: 0 minutes

Ingredients:

- 1 cup mixed berries (strawberries, blueberries, raspberries)
- 1/2 cup Greek yogurt
- 1/2 cup almond milk
- 2 tablespoons collagen powder
- 1 tablespoon honey (optional)
- Ice cubes

Instructions:

1. Combine all ingredients in a blender.
2. Blend until smooth.
3. Add ice cubes and blend again for a refreshing texture.
4. Serve immediately.

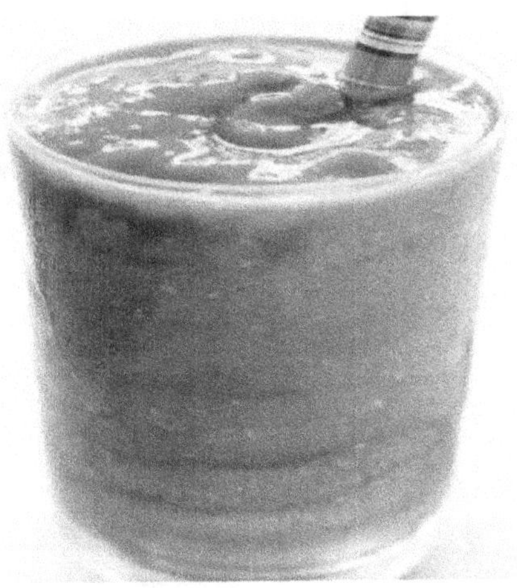

5. **Pomegranate and Acai Superfood Smoothie**

Description: A superfood-rich smoothie full of antioxidants to support heart health and overall vitality.

Serving Size: 2 servings

Prep Time: 10 minutes

Cooking Time: 0 minutes

Ingredients:

- 1 cup pomegranate juice
- 1 packet of frozen acai puree
- 1/2 cup mixed berries (blueberries, raspberries)
- 1/2 banana
- 1/2 cup almond milk

Instructions:

1. Combine all ingredients in a blender.
2. Blend until smooth and creamy.
3. Serve immediately.

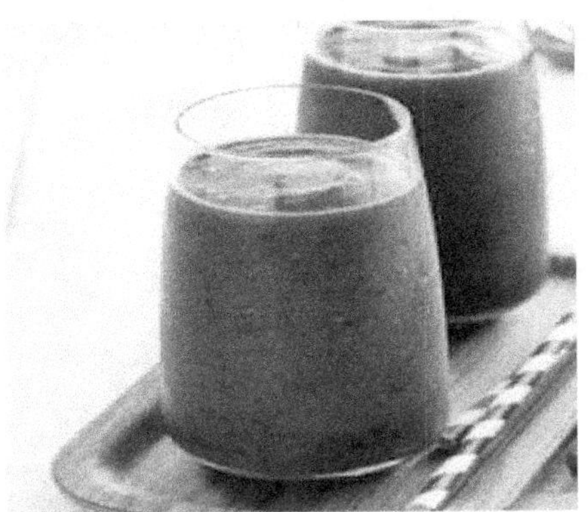

These recipes offer a range of beverages rich in nutrients and antioxidants, promoting ageless wellness and supporting a healthy lifestyle. Enjoy!

Incorporating Super Drinks into Your Daily Routine

Super drinks are made with superfoods, which are extremely potent and offer a host of health advantages. Superfoods include things like maca, cocoa, spirulina, and matcha. Antioxidants, vitamins, minerals, and phytonutrients found in abundance in these superfoods promote general health, energy levels, and immunological function.

Adding super drinks to your morning tea or coffee is a simple way to include them into your daily routine. For an energy and mental clarity boost, try mixing a scoop of matcha powder into your morning latte. Superfoods may also be blended into juices or smoothies to add even more nutrients.

1. Morning Energy Booster: Matcha Latte

Description: Start your day with a burst of natural energy from matcha green tea, rich in antioxidants.

Serving Size: 1 serving

Prep Time: 5 minutes

Cooking Time: 5 minutes

Ingredients:

- 1 teaspoon matcha green tea powder
- 1 cup almond milk (or milk of choice)
- 1 tablespoon honey (adjust to taste)

Instructions:

1. In a small saucepan, warm the almond milk but do not boil.
2. In a cup, whisk matcha powder and honey with a small amount of hot water until smooth.
3. Pour the warm milk over the matcha mixture and stir well.
4. Enjoy your matcha latte.

2. Afternoon Immunity Booster: Turmeric Golden Milk

Description: Boost your immune system with this soothing and anti-inflammatory turmeric drink.

Serving Size: 1 serving

Prep Time: 5 minutes

Cooking Time: 10 minutes

Ingredients:

- 1 cup milk (dairy or non-dairy)
- 1/2 teaspoon ground turmeric
- 1/4 teaspoon ground black pepper
- 1/2 teaspoon honey (adjust to taste)
- 1/4 teaspoon ground cinnamon (optional)

Instructions:

1. In a small saucepan, whisk together milk, turmeric, black pepper, and honey.
2. Heat the mixture on low-medium heat for about 10 minutes, stirring constantly.
3. Add cinnamon if desired, and enjoy your golden milk.

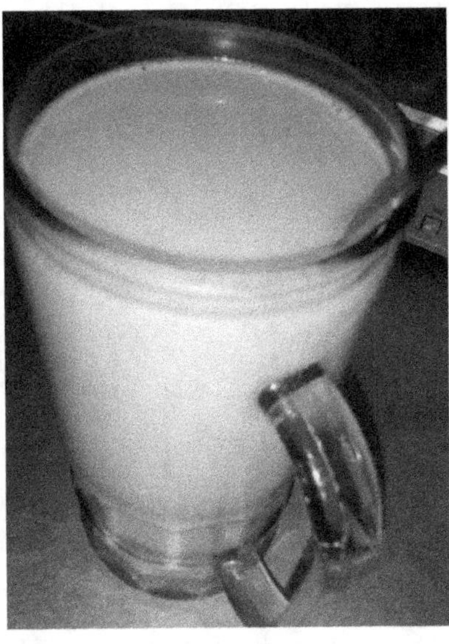

3. **Pre-Workout Fuel: Beet and Berry Smoothie**

Description: A nutritious smoothie with beets and berries to provide sustained energy for your workout.

Serving Size: 1 serving

Prep Time: 5 minutes

Cooking Time: 0 minutes

Ingredients:

- 1 small cooked beet, peeled and diced
- 1/2 cup mixed berries (strawberries, blueberries, raspberries)
- 1/2 banana
- 1/2 cup Greek yogurt
- 1/2 cup almond milk
- 1 tablespoon honey (optional)

Instructions:

1. Combine all ingredients in a blender.
2. Blend until smooth and creamy.
3. Enjoy your pre-workout beet and berry smoothie.

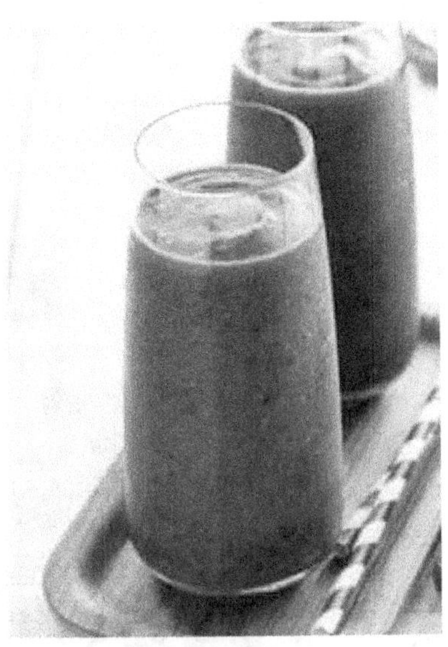

4. Digestive Health Elixir: Apple Cider Vinegar Tonic

Description: A tonic with apple cider vinegar to aid digestion and promote gut health.

Serving Size: 1 serving

Prep Time: 2 minutes

Cooking Time: 0 minutes

Ingredients:

- 1 tablespoon raw, unfiltered apple cider vinegar
- 1 cup water
- 1 teaspoon honey (adjust to taste)
- A squeeze of lemon juice

Instructions:

1. Mix apple cider vinegar, water, honey, and lemon juice in a glass.
2. Stir well and drink before or after meals for digestive support.

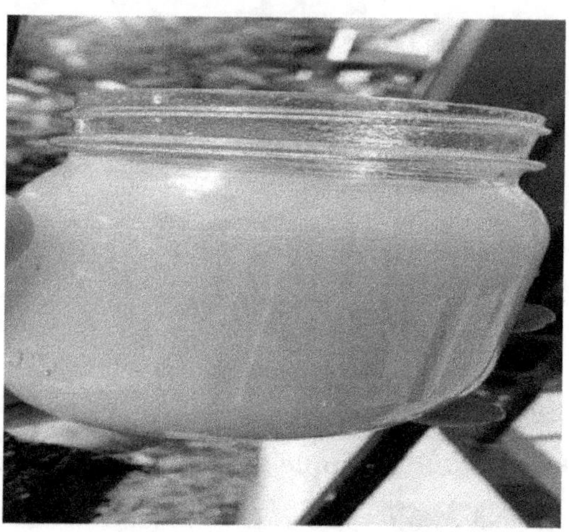

5. Evening Calm and Relaxation: Chamomile Tea

Description: Wind down with a cup of chamomile tea, known for its calming properties.

Serving Size: 1 serving

Prep Time: 5 minutes

Cooking Time: 5 minutes

Ingredients:

- 1 chamomile tea bag

- 1 cup boiling water
- 1 teaspoon honey (adjust to taste)
- A slice of lemon (optional)

Instructions:

1. Place the chamomile tea bag in a cup.
2. Pour boiling water over the tea bag and let steep for 5 minutes.
3. Add honey and a slice of lemon if desired.
4. Enjoy your soothing chamomile tea.

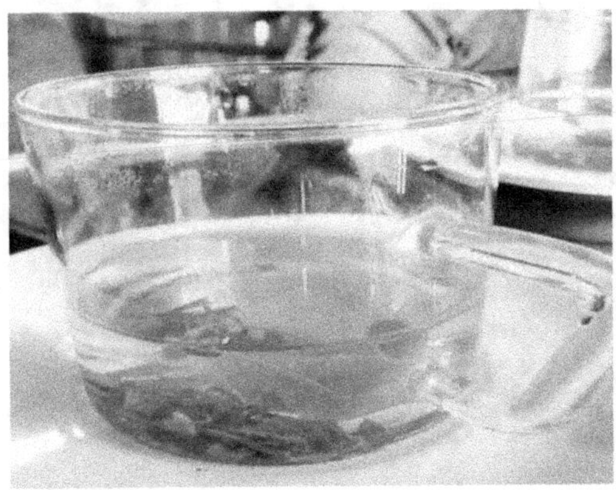

Incorporating these super drinks into your daily routine can provide various health benefits and make your day more enjoyable. Enjoy the benefits of these delicious and nutritious beverages

To sum up, selecting nutrient-dense and hydrating drinks such as smoothies, juices, and elixirs may help maintain ageless wellbeing and encourage radiant health. Adding super drinks to your daily routine is a simple way to improve your consumption of superfoods and take advantage of their potent nutrients. To your health, cheers!

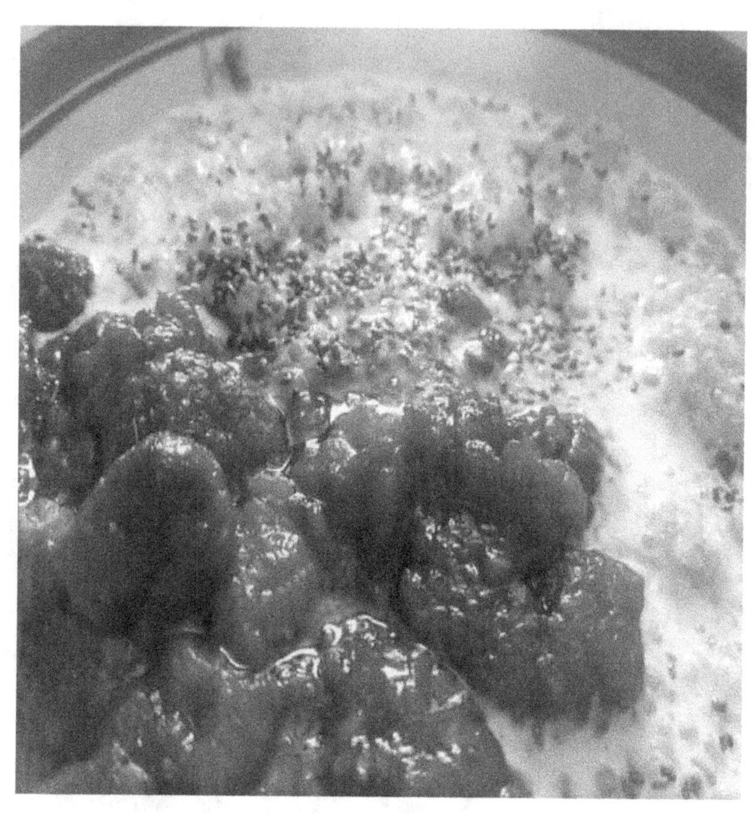

Chapter Nine

A Lifestyle of Forever Strength

Greetings and welcome to "A Lifestyle of Forever Strength," where we will be starting the last phase of our quest to discover the keys to living a young, energetic life. We explore the holistic approach to wellbeing in this chapter, emphasizing the relationship between exercise, food, and mindfulness. Here you'll find long-term maintenance techniques for a young appearance as well as priceless advice for eternal strength.

Balancing Diet with Exercise and Mindfulness

A healthy lifestyle necessitates a balance between regular exercise, a nutritious diet, and mindfulness exercises. You may get maximum health and wellness by implementing all three into your everyday regimen.

1. Diet: Fueling Your Body for Success

A balanced diet is the cornerstone of any healthy lifestyle. It provides the essential nutrients your body needs to function optimally. It's not about following the latest fad diet but rather adopting a sustainable eating plan. Focus on:

- Whole Foods: Incorporate plenty of fruits, vegetables, whole grains, and lean proteins into your diet. These foods are rich in essential vitamins and minerals.
- Portion Control: Be mindful of portion sizes to avoid overeating. Listen to your body's hunger and fullness cues.
- Hydration: Stay properly hydrated by drinking enough water throughout the day. It's crucial for digestion and overall well-being.

2. Exercise: The Key to Physical Vitality

Exercise is the perfect complement to a balanced diet. Regular physical activity offers a multitude of benefits, including:

- Weight Management: It helps you maintain a healthy weight or reach your weight loss goals.
- Strength and Endurance: Builds muscle and cardiovascular endurance, making daily activities easier.
- Mental Health: Exercise releases endorphins, reducing stress and enhancing mood.
- Improved Sleep: Regular physical activity can lead to better sleep, which is vital for overall well-being.

3. Mindfulness: Nurturing Your Mental Health

Incorporating mindfulness into your daily routine can have a profound impact on your mental and emotional well-being. Mindfulness practices include:

- Meditation: Taking time each day to meditate can help reduce stress, improve focus, and increase self-awareness.
- Yoga: Yoga combines physical postures with breath control and meditation. It's a fantastic way to reduce stress and improve flexibility.
- Mindful Eating: Paying attention to what and how you eat can prevent overeating and promote a healthier relationship with food.

4. Finding Balance

Balancing diet, exercise, and mindfulness is about finding equilibrium in your life. It's not about perfection but about progress. Here are some tips for achieving this balance:

- Create a Routine: Establish a daily or weekly schedule that includes time for exercise, meal planning, and mindfulness practices.
- Set Realistic Goals: Ensure your goals are achievable and sustainable. Small, gradual changes are often more successful than drastic ones.

- Listen to Your Body: Pay attention to how your body feels, both physically and mentally. Adapt your approach based on your needs.
- Seek Support: Don't hesitate to seek guidance from healthcare professionals, nutritionists, or personal trainers if needed.

Strategies for Maintaining a Youthful Appearance

Unlocking the secrets to maintaining a youthful appearance is a pursuit as old as time itself. In this quest, we seek not the mythical Fountain of Youth, but rather a harmonious blend of science, lifestyle choices, and mindful practices. The strategies we explore in this chapter are grounded in the belief that age is just a number and that a vibrant, youthful appearance can be preserved and even enhanced.

The Importance of Proper Nutrition

You must eat a balanced diet in order to provide your body the nutrients it needs in order to function correctly. Make an effort to include entire foods in your meals, such as fruits, vegetables, whole grains, lean meats, and healthy fats. Steer clear of processed and sugary meals at all costs.

Making good food choices all day long may be ensured by organizing and preparing your meals. To maintain a steady metabolism and energy levels, try to consume three well-balanced meals and two snacks each day.

The Advantages of Regular Exercises

Maintaining a healthy weight, enhancing cardiovascular health, and lowering the risk of chronic illnesses like diabetes and cancer all depend on exercise. Make an enjoyable hobby or pastime a regular part of your day. This might be anything from weightlifting, yoga, riding, swimming, or strolling.

If you have trouble staying motivated, think about hiring a personal trainer or enrolling in a fitness class to help. Five days a week, try to get in at least 30 minutes of moderate-intensity activity each day.

The Power of Mindfulness Practices

Deep breathing exercises, yoga, and meditation are examples of mindfulness techniques that can lower stress, enhance mental clarity, and enhance general wellbeing. Include these routines in your everyday life to assist with stress and anxiety management.

Begin by dedicating a short period of time each day to deep breathing techniques or meditation. Another option is to attempt a yoga class or use internet tools to practice at home.

Finding the Right Balance

It might be difficult to strike a balance between a healthy diet, consistent exercise, and mindfulness exercises, but doing so is crucial to reaching optimal health and wellbeing. Set modest initial targets for yourself and work your way up to include these routines in your everyday life.

Keep in mind that each person's path is different, and what suits one person might not suit another. Pay attention to your body and figure out what suits you the best. You may have a balanced and healthful lifestyle if you are committed to it and act consistently.

Strategies for Maintaining a Youthful Appearance

The quest to discover the keys of keeping one's appearance young is as old as time itself. Instead of the fabled Fountain of Youth, we want to find a harmonic fusion of science, lifestyle decisions, and introspective activities. The techniques we discuss in this chapter are based on the idea that youth is only a number and that it is possible to maintain and even improve a lively, young appearance.

The Science of Producing Collagen

Often called the scaffolding of the body, collagen is essential to young skin. Its natural reduction in production with time causes sagging and wrinkles. We may, however, delay this process by adopting lifestyle choices and dietary choices that are high in substances that enhance collagen production. Discover how to preserve the suppleness of your skin and maximize the benefits of collagen.

The Craft of Beauty Rituals

Our skin is our canvas, and keeping a young glow depends greatly on how we take care of it. Learn the art of creating skincare regimens that work for your particular skin type and requirements. We reveal the crucial components that maintain the brightness of your skin, from caring for your skin on a regular basis to the need for sun protection.

The Beauty of Hydration

A well-hydrated body is a hallmark of youth. Dehydration can lead to dull and tired-looking skin, so staying adequately hydrated is vital. Learn the secrets of proper hydration and how water, along with specific hydrating foods, can keep your skin plump and glowing.

Embracing Holistic Wellness

A youthful appearance isn't just skin deep; it's a reflection of your overall well-being. We explore the importance of balancing your mental and physical health. Stress, in particular, can accelerate the aging process. Discover mindfulness and stress-reduction techniques that not only promote inner calm but also reflect on your outward appearance.

The Synergy of Diet and Skincare

The connection between your diet and the health of your skin is profound. Explore the nutrient-rich foods that serve as natural beauty elixirs. Learn how antioxidants, vitamins, and minerals can enhance your skin's texture and complexion. We also delve into the importance of healthy fats and their role in maintaining skin elasticity.

In the pursuit of a youthful appearance, science and artistry come together to form a dynamic partnership. With strategies deeply rooted in the principles of self-care, we embark on a journey where age is a mere number, and your appearance reflects the vibrancy within. These strategies empower you to face each day with confidence, knowing that you have the tools to maintain a youthful and radiant visage.

Tips on Staying Forever Strong in the Long Term

The desire to maintain strength, health, and vibrancy as we age is something that all people strive for. The path to long-lasting strength is a lifetime endeavor rather than just a few moments of well-being. This chapter covers practical advice and long-term techniques for preserving your health and vigor. These are not just for today, but also for the coming years, decades, and beyond.

Consistency is Key

Consistency is one of the most important rules for being powerful forever. Be consistent and sensible in your lifestyle decisions. Enduring vitality is based on a well-rounded diet, regular exercise, and a conscious attitude to stress management. It's about making a consistent daily commitment to your health rather than making short, strong spurts of effort.

Personalized Fitness Routines

Since no two people are alike, their fitness requirements are also unique. Make a customized exercise program that takes into account your body's preferences, limitations, and strengths. Think about combining aerobic, strength, flexibility, and balancing workouts. Over time, your body will appreciate the effort.

Mindful Nutrition Choices
Your health now will be greatly impacted by the meals you choose to eat tomorrow. Adopt a diet full of whole, nutrient-dense meals to provide you long-lasting energy and sustenance. Give lean proteins, whole grains, fruits, veggies, and healthy fats first priority. A well-balanced diet is frequently indicated by a colorful plate.

Stay Curious and Continue Learning
There is an intellectual component to the pursuit of lifetime strength. Continue your curiosity and education about aging, wellness, and health. Investigate fresh methods for mindfulness, fitness, and nutrition. Your ability to adjust to your body's and mind's shifting requirements will improve as you gain more knowledge.

Mindfulness and Stress Reduction
Stress is a quiet but deadly enemy of long-term resilience and well-being. Practice awareness by using techniques like deep breathing, meditation, and relaxation. By lowering stress and promoting mental clarity, these techniques increase general wellbeing.

Build a Supportive Community
A network of dependable connections is a powerful source of energy. Maintain relationships with loved ones, close friends, and those who share your dedication to long-term heath. In addition to providing inspiration, a caring community promotes mental health.

Celebrate Achievements, Big and Small
Lastly, whether they are little successes or significant turning points, take some time to enjoy your accomplishments. Acknowledge and treat yourself for your dedication to your long-term health and well-being. These festivities act as a reminder of the strides you've made along the way.
It's not about short fixes or stopgap measures in the quest for eternal strength. It involves piecing together decisions that are balanced, sustainable, and sensitive to your particular circumstances. These

pointers offer a road map for continuing to be strong forever, and as you follow it, you'll discover that strength genuinely knows no age.

Chapter Ten

Beyond the Kitchen - Tips and Tricks

In this last chapter, we go outside the kitchen to explore a realm of useful knowledge that guarantees a smooth and long-lasting transition to timeless nutrition. "Beyond the Kitchen - Tips and Tricks" is a goldmine of insightful guidance drawn from both seasoned nutrition professionals and hobbyists. Here, we delve into the fine art of grocery shopping and ingredient sourcing, reveal the insider tips for effective food storage, and unearth creative tricks for meal planning. Additionally, we include the inspiring testimonies and triumphant tales of readers just like you who have started on their own transforming paths to perpetual health and vigor.

Practical Advice for Grocery Shopping and Ingredient Sourcing

It is frequently reminiscent of going on a gastronomic excursion to browse the aisles of a grocery shop. In this area, we provide helpful guidance to help you choose foods and grocery shops in a thoughtful, health-conscious manner. This is where your quest to ageless nutrition starts—within the shop.

Shop with Purpose

Bring a shopping list with you before you enter the store. This small deed might have a big impact on your shopping choices. Having a well-planned list helps you stay on course and guarantees that you will have the components needed to prepare healthful, well-balanced meals. It's a tool that helps you maintain your long-term dedication to wellness.

Figuring Out Food Labels

Deciphering food labels is one of the most useful skills you can learn. Acquire the ability to differentiate between promotional platitudes and actual nutritional value. Keep a careful eye on ingredient lists, portion sizes, and macronutrient counts. Whether your goal is to improve your consumption of a certain nutrient or find items with fewer chemicals, having this knowledge empowers you to make wise decisions.

Fresh, Seasonal and Local

When procuring ingredients, give top priority to seasonal, local, and fresh vegetables. In addition to having higher flavor and nutritional content, these foods also help to support local farmers and businesses, which helps to create a more sustainable food system. For fresh, locally grown goodies, check out farmers' markets or think about signing up for a community-supported agriculture (CSA) program.

Organic and GMO Options

Selecting organic and non-GMO (genetically modified organism) items can help reduce your exposure to synthetic chemicals and pesticides, while it's not always necessary. When making purchases, exercise caution and choose non-GMO options wherever available, as well as organic food that is on the "Dirty Dozen" list (a list of fruits and vegetables with the highest pesticide levels).

Cost-conscious Purchasing

Maintaining a healthy diet doesn't have to break the bank. Seek out retail brands, special offers, and discounts that provide premium ingredients at more reasonable costs. To cut costs, think about buying some products in bulk, such as whole grains. Long-term financial savings and a decrease in food waste may both be achieved with meal planning.

Be Mindful of Food Allergies and Sensitivities

If you have dietary sensitivities or allergies, it's important to read labels carefully and look into substitute goods. Thankfully, most retailers now provide a growing selection of gluten-free and allergy-friendly alternatives. Keeping an eye out for the source of ingredients is essential to protecting your health.

The decisions you make at the grocery store set the course for your quest toward timeless nutrition. Equipped with useful guidance, a well organized shopping list, and a comprehension of food labels, you may convert your grocery shopping encounter into a vibrant manifestation of your dedication to well-being and energy. Every shopping trip turns into an opportunity to take care of your body, give back to the community, and start down the path to a lifetime of wellbeing.

Food Storage and Meal Planning Hacks

Effectiveness in the kitchen is crucial to sustaining a classic and dynamic diet. Meal planning and efficient food storage are the first steps in this process. This section contains a number of clever tips that can not only prolong the freshness of your food but also simplify the process of meal planning and preparation.

Increase Shelf Life through Careful Storage

1. Mason Jar Wonders: Mason jars hold more than just pickles and jams. You may store grains, nuts, dried fruits, and even salads in them. They create an aesthetically pleasing pantry and their airtight sealing keeps items fresh.
2. Fresh herbs should be frozen to prevent wilting in the refrigerator. Chop them, toss with olive oil, then put in ice cube trays to freeze. You may easily add a herb cube to your food whenever you need a taste boost.
3. Fruit Preservation: Use airtight containers for berries and breathable bags for lettuce and other greens to keep fruit fresher for longer. Additionally, think about spending money on vegetable storage bags that can absorb extra moisture.
4. Egg-cellent Storage: You might be surprised to learn how long eggs can last. Keep them in the coldest section of your refrigerator, still in their original box. They are shielded from moisture and smells by the container.

Simplify Meal Preparation

1. Combined Cooking: Set aside a day for cooking in bulk. Make more of the staple foods, such as grilled chicken, rice, and beans. These might be the basis for a number of dinners that you prepare over the week.
2. Meal Prep Dishes: Purchase a set of premium meal prep containers with several sections. This keeps your lunches organized and simplifies meal portioning.
3. Rotate your recipes in your meal plan to stay away from boredom. Assign daily meals to particular days of the week to simplify grocery list planning and guarantee a well-rounded diet.
4. Shopping Lists with a Goal: When creating your shopping list, specify the amounts and purposes you'll need. By doing this, you guarantee that you only buy what you need and reduce waste.
5. Clever Remainders: Make meal plans that include leftovers. You may use these to make new recipes, which will save you time and cut down on food waste.

The Freezer's Power

1. Freeze Any Oversight: Freeze leftovers instead of throwing them out. Invest in sealed containers, date them, and savor less expensive and healthier homemade "TV dinners"
2. Fresh Herbs in Ice: You may freeze fresh herbs in olive oil in ice cube trays, just like you would with herb cubes. This increases their shelf life so you may always have fresh tastes in your meals.
3. Fruit Smoothies: Prepare your preferred smoothie ingredients in advance, put them into bags, and then freeze them. In this manner, when you're ready for a quick and wholesome breakfast, you can just combine them with a drink.

You may reduce food waste, save time and money, and integrate healthy eating into your daily life by learning meal planning and food storage tips. By following these useful suggestions, you may take use of fresher ingredients, a well-organized kitchen, and the convenience of pre-planned meals, all contributing to your journey toward timeless nutrition.

Conclusion

By the time you finish the "Forever Strong Cookbook," you will have traveled a long way across the domains of health, vitality, and nutrition. This cookbook is a guide to adopting age-defying nutrition and making a lifetime commitment to your well-being, not just a compilation of recipes. Let's review the most important lessons learned, provide support for your further path, and exchange helpful materials and acknowledgements.

You have studied the principles of nutrition that defies aging, learned how eating affects aging, and examined the functions of antioxidants, nutrients, and superfoods throughout this cookbook. You've prepared gorgeous dinners, well-balanced lunches, and nutrient-dense breakfasts. You've perfected healthy and palate-pleasing appetizers, sides, and desserts. You now know useful advice for meal planning, grocery shopping, and locating ingredients. Reader testimonies and success stories that highlight the life-changing potential of making health-conscious decisions have motivated you. These essential learnings serve as the cornerstones of your enduring path toward timeless nourishment.

This is only the beginning of your lifelong journey toward optimal health and energy. Accept this obligation with zeal and diligence. Always keep in mind that tiny, regular improvements result in long-lasting effects and that every meal is an opportunity to nurture your body. Aim for harmony in your selections and relish the bright tastes of wholesome meals. It is within your power to stay young-looking, strong, and healthy for the rest of your life. Treat your body with love and respect since it is your everlasting friend.

Check out the links and other reading suggestions in the appendix to carry on your search for nutrition that defies age. These resources provide in-depth knowledge, direction, and motivation for your travels. We also want to express our sincere appreciation to all of the readers and professionals who helped to make this cookbook. Your suggestions, anecdotes, and knowledge have enhanced our project and made it a genuinely team effort.

You have the resources, information, and motivation to dedicate your life to your health as you set out on your path to age-defying nutrition. More than just a cookbook, the "Forever Strong Cookbook" is your amazing guide to a happier, healthier, and more fulfilled existence. I hope that your experience serves as a witness to the incredible power of taking care of your body, mind, and spirit.

Appendix

You'll find a plethora of extra knowledge and resources to further your culinary and nutritional exploration in the "Forever Strong Cookbook" appendix. This part is intended to help you comprehend nutritional information. It includes an index for easy and rapid recipe retrieval, a glossary of important phrases, conversion tables, and measures for accuracy in your cooking.

Nutritional Information and Glossary

When it comes to nutrition that defies age, information truly is power. Knowing what nutrients are in the food you eat gives you the power to make wise, health-conscious decisions. In addition to offering tasty recipes, the "Forever Strong Cookbook" is a helpful tool for understanding the nutritional content of your meals. We've included a glossary of key words and nutritional facts here to help you on your path to lifetime vitality.

Nutritional Information

1. Learn about the three main macronutrients: lipids, proteins, and carbs. Learn about their functions in your diet and how to balance them for the best possible health.
2. Explore the realm of micronutrients, encompassing vitamins and minerals. Recognize their benefits to your health and where to locate them in your food.
3. Caloric Values: Learn how many calories are in different foods to better control how much energy you take in and use.
4. Dietary Fiber: Learn about the advantages of dietary fiber, how it affects satiety and digestion, and how to include it in your regular meals.
5. Sugars: Know the difference between added and natural sugars. Learn where hidden sugars come from and how to cut back on your intake.

6. Sodium: Recognize the function of sodium in your diet, how to control your salt consumption, and the possible health risks.

Glossary

1. Discover the realm of antioxidants, which are compounds that help shield your body from the aging process and the harmful impacts of free radicals.
2. Superfoods: Find out how to include these nutrient-dense powerhouses into your diet as well as about their remarkable health benefits.
3. Glycemic Index: Recognize the importance of the glycemic index in controlling blood sugar levels and general health.
4. Learn the significance of omega-3 fatty acids for heart and brain health, as well as which foods are the finest suppliers of these essential fats.
5. Crucial Elements: Learn about the vitamins and minerals that are necessary for different body processes, as well as critical nutrients and how to make sure you get enough of them.
6. Examine the idea of bioavailability, which refers to the extent to which the nutrients in the food you eat may be absorbed and used by your body.
7. Dietary standards: To assist you in maintaining a balanced and health-conscious diet, familiarize yourself with suggested daily allowances and dietary standards.

With this terminology and nutritional information at your disposal, you can make wise, health-conscious decisions when exploring other cuisines. You are equipped with the knowledge and skills to interpret the nutritional value of your food and make sure that each mouthful fulfills your lifelong goal of vitality and well-being.

Conversion Charts and Measurements

Accuracy is critical when it comes to fine dining and healthy eating. The goal of the "Forever Strong Cookbook" is to improve your cooking abilities and uphold your lifetime dedication to age-defying nutrition. This area contains conversion tables and measurements—a virtual toolbox with vital information to guarantee that your recipes are always exceptional.

Conversion Charts:

1. Learn how to convert quantities between teaspoons and gallons so that you can measure liquids precisely for your recipes.
2. Weight Measurements: These weight conversions, which go from ounces to grams and pounds to kilograms, guarantee that your components are weighed precisely.
3. Temperature Conversions: When working with temperature-sensitive culinary methods, knowing how to convert between Fahrenheit and Celsius is crucial.
4. Conversions from Cup to Gram: Recipes frequently use cups as the measurement unit; this chart allows you to convert cups to grams for a variety of substances, such as flour and sugar.

Index for Quick Recipe Retrieval

Maintaining an age-defying nutritional lifestyle requires efficiency in the kitchen. The "Forever Strong Cookbook" has been carefully arranged to make cooking easier for you. An easy-to-use method to quickly discover your favorite recipes based on categories, courses, or dietary requirements may be found in this index.

By Category:

1. Breakfasts: A selection of wholesome breakfast dishes to get you through the morning.
2. Lunches: healthy, filling, and energizing midday meals that keep you going throughout the day.
3. Dinners: Tasty, health-conscious evening meals that come with dietary restrictions and unique recipes for parties and get-togethers.
4. Snacks & Sides: mouthwatering, nutrient-dense snacks for long-lasting energy, as well as side dishes that go well with your main courses and options for different diets.
5. Desserts: An assortment of decadent and healthful desserts, along with recipes to fulfill your sweet appetite guilt-free, including sugar-free and allergy-friendly alternatives.

By Course

1. Appetizers Delicious appetizers that entice your palate before the main entrée.
2. Main Dishes: filling meals that form the basis of your dinner.
3. Side dishes: Enhance your meal experience with complimentary dishes.
4. Desserts: Whether decadent or health-conscious, these sweet finishes defy aging.

By Preference

1. Vegan Recipes: Plant-based dishes that complement a vegan diet.
2. Low-Carb Recipes: Recipes created by fans of low-carb cuisine.
3. Recipes that are gluten-free: Foods suitable for a gluten-free diet.
4. Recipes that are high in nutrients: Recipes that are designed to be highly nutritious.
5. Recipes that are quick and easy to prepare—meals that are perfect for people on the run.

Finding your favorite recipes is made easier with this index, which also makes meal preparation and planning a snap. Whether you're craving a substantial breakfast, a well-balanced lunch, a sophisticated supper, or a decadent dessert, this index guarantees that your culinary adventure will be both easy and satisfying.

Recap of Key Takeaways

By reading this Book, you've taken a wonderful step toward adopting the concepts of diet that defies aging and lifelong vitality. Let's review the main points that sum up this cookbook's essence and provide you the tools you need to achieve long-lasting wellbeing as we come to an end with this culinary adventure.

1. The Fundamentals of Nutrition to Combat Aging: You now know the fundamentals of nutrition that defies age and the critical role that diet plays in preserving a young, energetic life.
2. Impact of nutrition on Aging: You've discovered the keys to fueling your body for long-lasting vigor and wellbeing by investigating the significant effects of nutrition on the aging process.
3. Function of Antioxidants, Nutrients, and Superfoods: You have made it a daily habit to include antioxidants, vital nutrients, and superfoods in your diet to strengthen your body against the ravages of aging.
4. Meals That Are Both Balanced and Satisfying: You now know how to prepare meals that are both nutrient-rich and satisfying to the taste senses and your body.
5. Efficiency in Food Storage and Meal Planning: You've made the effort of adhering to a health-conscious diet easier by learning the art of effective food storage and thoughtful meal planning.
6. Reader Testimonials that Transform: The motivational success stories and reader testimonials have demonstrated the transformational power of age-defying nutrition, demonstrating how a dedication to health can result in amazing transformations in all facets of life.

7. Accept a Lifetime Promise: This is only the start of a lifelong adventure that is dedicated to your well-being. Nutrition that defies age is a journey, not a destination.
8. Important Sources & Additional Reading: Examine the helpful links and other reading suggestions in the appendix to carry on with your pursuit of vitality and health.

Each of these takeaways represents a pillar of strength in your journey towards timeless nutrition. Together, they form the foundation of a lifestyle that defies the limitations of age and promises enduring well-being. With this knowledge, you are empowered to make informed, health-conscious choices every day and embrace a life of radiant health and vitality.

Encouragement for a Lifelong Commitment to Age-Defying Nutrition

As you close the pages of the "Forever Strong Cookbook," you stand at the threshold of a transformative journey towards age-defying nutrition and lifelong wellness. While the cookbook has imparted invaluable knowledge and delicious recipes, the journey ahead is an enduring commitment to your well-being. Here's some heartfelt encouragement to inspire you on this lifelong path:

1. Honor Progress, Not Perfection: Keep in mind that nobody is flawless and that following strict guidelines won't help you on your path. No matter how tiny the advancement you make along the road, acknowledge it. Every decision that prioritizes health is a positive step.
2. Modest Amounts, Huge Effect: Age-defying diet is about incremental, consistent improvements made over time rather than big, abrupt overhauls. Every nourishing meal and conscientious decision you make adds to your long-lasting health.

3. Love Your Body: Show your body the respect it deserves and take good care of it throughout your life. Your body is traveling with you, so treat it with compassion and respect.

4. Various and Tasty Options: Maintaining an age-defying diet may be a tasty and enjoyable experience. Accept the variety of flavors, meals, and culinary traditions. Taste foreign foods, experiment with new recipes, and keep your meals interesting.

5. Age-defying nutrition is based mostly on the practice of mindful eating. Enjoy every mouthful, be mindful of your body's signals of hunger and fullness, and stay in the present. It concerns how you eat as much as what you consume.

6. Community and Support: Share your adventure with like-minded people and enlist their assistance. One of the most effective motivators might be a supportive community. Be an inspiration to others, seek help, and share your triumphs with others.

7. Keep Yourself Inquisitive and Curious: Keep learning about wellness, health, and nutrition. Remain observant and inquisitive about novel discoveries and methodologies. Your level of empowerment increases with your knowledge.

8. Accept the Journey: Keep in mind that this is a way of life rather than a destination. Accept it wholeheartedly because eating a diet that defies aging is a lifetime commitment to your health and vigor.

9. Prioritize Self-Care: For your mental and emotional health, give self-care a higher priority than diet. A healthy existence requires self-compassion, mindfulness, and stress management.

10. You Will Always Be Powerful: Above all, remember that you possess the knowledge, willpower, and fortitude to dedicate your entire life to an age-defying diet. Your trip is evidence of your ongoing vitality and your unwavering strength.

With this encouragement, step boldly into the path of age-defying nutrition. Your journey is a remarkable adventure of lifelong wellness, resilience, and the art of embracing age with grace. Every day is an opportunity to nourish your body, rejuvenate your spirit, and become a living testament to the power of health-conscious choices.

Resources, Further Reading, and Acknowledgments

In your pursuit of age-defying nutrition and lifelong vitality through the "Forever Strong Cookbook," we want to ensure that your journey is enriched and your knowledge continually deepened. This section of resources, further reading recommendations, and acknowledgments is designed to provide you with the tools and inspiration to continue your quest for health and wellness.

Resources for Your Journey

- Cooking and Nutrition Classes: Consider enrolling in cooking and nutrition classes to enhance your culinary skills and deepen your understanding of age-defying nutrition.
- Online Communities: Join online communities, forums, and social media groups dedicated to healthy living. They provide a wealth of information and a supportive network of individuals on similar journeys.
- Cooking Apps: Explore cooking apps that offer a multitude of healthy recipes and meal planning tools, making it easier to embrace age-defying nutrition in your daily life.
- Nutrition Apps: Utilize nutrition apps to track your daily intake, monitor your progress, and receive personalized recommendations for a well-balanced diet.

Further Reading Recommendations

- "How Not to Die" by Dr. Michael Greger: This book explores the role of nutrition in preventing and reversing the most common chronic diseases, offering valuable insights for age-defying nutrition.

- "In Defense of Food" by Michael Pollan: Michael Pollan's exploration of the Western diet and the power of returning to traditional, real food is a thought-provoking read.
- "The Longevity Diet" by Valter Longo: Dr. Valter Longo delves into the science of aging and offers a comprehensive guide to nutrition and its role in promoting longevity.
- "The Blue Zones Kitchen" by Dan Buettner: This book explores the eating habits of people living in Blue Zones—areas known for exceptional longevity—and offers recipes that align with their dietary patterns.
- Academic Journals and Research Papers: For a deep dive into the science of nutrition, explore academic journals and research papers on topics related to age-defying nutrition and longevity.

Acknowledgments

The creation of the "Forever Strong Cookbook" would not have been possible without the collective effort and support of many individuals. We extend our sincere gratitude to:

- Our Readers: Your curiosity, feedback, and unwavering dedication to health have been the driving force behind this cookbook.
- Contributing Experts: We are grateful to the experts in the fields of nutrition, health, and wellness who provided their valuable insights and guidance.
- Friends and Family: To those who stood by us with encouragement, understanding, and countless taste tests, thank you for your unwavering support.
- Our Creative Team: The artists, designers, editors, and everyone involved in bringing this cookbook to life—thank you for your dedication and talent.
- Acknowledgment of Sources: We've drawn knowledge and inspiration from various sources, including books, research papers, and culinary traditions. We acknowledge and appreciate the wisdom shared by these sources.

Your contribution, support, and collaboration have been the pillars of this project. As we conclude this cookbook, we look forward to the shared journey of age-defying nutrition, well-being, and vitality. Thank you for being an integral part of our mission to inspire healthier and more vibrant lives.

FOREVER STRONG COOKBOOK
MEAL PLANNER

SUNDAY	BREAKFAST	
	LUNCH	
	DINNER	
MONDAY	BREAKFAST	
	LUNCH	
	DINNER	
TUESDAY	BREAKFAST	
	LUNCH	
	DINNER	
WEDNESDAY	BREAKFAST	
	LUNCH	
	DINNER	
THURSDAY	BREAKFAST	
	LUNCH	
	DINNER	
FRIDAY	BREAKFAST	
	LUNCH	
	DINNER	
SATURDAY	BREAKFAST	
	LUNCH	
	DINNER	

GROCERY LIST

SNACKS

FOREVER STRONG COOKBOOK
MEAL PLANNER

SUNDAY	BREAKFAST	
	LUNCH	
	DINNER	
MONDAY	BREAKFAST	
	LUNCH	
	DINNER	
TUESDAY	BREAKFAST	
	LUNCH	
	DINNER	
WEDNESDAY	BREAKFAST	
	LUNCH	
	DINNER	
THURSDAY	BREAKFAST	
	LUNCH	
	DINNER	
FRIDAY	BREAKFAST	
	LUNCH	
	DINNER	
SATURDAY	BREAKFAST	
	LUNCH	
	DINNER	

GROCERY LIST

SNACKS

FOREVER STRONG COOKBOOK
MEAL PLANNER

SUNDAY	BREAKFAST	
	LUNCH	
	DINNER	
MONDAY	BREAKFAST	
	LUNCH	
	DINNER	
TUESDAY	BREAKFAST	
	LUNCH	
	DINNER	
WEDNESDAY	BREAKFAST	
	LUNCH	
	DINNER	
THURSDAY	BREAKFAST	
	LUNCH	
	DINNER	
FRIDAY	BREAKFAST	
	LUNCH	
	DINNER	
SATURDAY	BREAKFAST	
	LUNCH	
	DINNER	

GROCERY LIST

SNACKS

FOREVER STRONG COOKBOOK MEAL PLANNER

SUNDAY	BREAKFAST	
	LUNCH	
	DINNER	
MONDAY	BREAKFAST	
	LUNCH	
	DINNER	
TUESDAY	BREAKFAST	
	LUNCH	
	DINNER	
WEDNESDAY	BREAKFAST	
	LUNCH	
	DINNER	
THURSDAY	BREAKFAST	
	LUNCH	
	DINNER	
FRIDAY	BREAKFAST	
	LUNCH	
	DINNER	
SATURDAY	BREAKFAST	
	LUNCH	
	DINNER	

GROCERY LIST

SNACKS

FOREVER STRONG COOKBOOK
MEAL PLANNER

SUNDAY	BREAKFAST	
	LUNCH	
	DINNER	
MONDAY	BREAKFAST	
	LUNCH	
	DINNER	
TUESDAY	BREAKFAST	
	LUNCH	
	DINNER	
WEDNESDAY	BREAKFAST	
	LUNCH	
	DINNER	
THURSDAY	BREAKFAST	
	LUNCH	
	DINNER	
FRIDAY	BREAKFAST	
	LUNCH	
	DINNER	
SATURDAY	BREAKFAST	
	LUNCH	
	DINNER	

GROCERY LIST

SNACKS

FOREVER STRONG COOKBOOK
MEAL PLANNER

SUNDAY	BREAKFAST	
	LUNCH	
	DINNER	
MONDAY	BREAKFAST	
	LUNCH	
	DINNER	
TUESDAY	BREAKFAST	
	LUNCH	
	DINNER	
WEDNESDAY	BREAKFAST	
	LUNCH	
	DINNER	
THURSDAY	BREAKFAST	
	LUNCH	
	DINNER	
FRIDAY	BREAKFAST	
	LUNCH	
	DINNER	
SATURDAY	BREAKFAST	
	LUNCH	
	DINNER	

GROCERY LIST

SNACKS

FOREVER STRONG COOKBOOK
MEAL PLANNER

SUNDAY	BREAKFAST	
	LUNCH	
	DINNER	

MONDAY	BREAKFAST	
	LUNCH	
	DINNER	

TUESDAY	BREAKFAST	
	LUNCH	
	DINNER	

WEDNESDAY	BREAKFAST	
	LUNCH	
	DINNER	

THURSDAY	BREAKFAST	
	LUNCH	
	DINNER	

FRIDAY	BREAKFAST	
	LUNCH	
	DINNER	

SATURDAY	BREAKFAST	
	LUNCH	
	DINNER	

GROCERY LIST

SNACKS

FOREVER STRONG COOKBOOK
MEAL PLANNER

SUNDAY	BREAKFAST	
	LUNCH	
	DINNER	
MONDAY	BREAKFAST	
	LUNCH	
	DINNER	
TUESDAY	BREAKFAST	
	LUNCH	
	DINNER	
WEDNESDAY	BREAKFAST	
	LUNCH	
	DINNER	
THURSDAY	BREAKFAST	
	LUNCH	
	DINNER	
FRIDAY	BREAKFAST	
	LUNCH	
	DINNER	
SATURDAY	BREAKFAST	
	LUNCH	
	DINNER	

GROCERY LIST

SNACKS